The State of Medicine

To my family, and especially my mum and husband who are unfailingly, uncomplainingly supportive of my work.

I owe you dozens of uninterrupted games of Catan, and lots of ironing.

Margaret McCartney

The State of Medicine
Keeping the promise of the NHS

The State of Medicine: Keeping the promise of the NHS

First published in the UK by Pinter & Martin Ltd 2016

Copyright © Margaret McCartney 2016

All rights reserved

ISBN 978-1-78066-400-2

Also available as an ebook

The right of Margaret McCartney to be identified as the author of this work has been asserted by her in accordance with the Copyright, Designs and Patent Act of 1988

Edited by Christopher Westhorp
Proofread by Chloe Pew Latter
Index by Helen Bilton

British Library Cataloguing-in-Publication Data
A catalogue record for this book is available from the British Library

Printed in Great Britain by Ashford Colour Press Ltd, Gosport, Hampshire

This book has been printed on paper that is sourced and harvested from sustainable forests and is FSC accredited

Pinter & Martin Ltd
6 Effra Parade
London SW2 1PS

pinterandmartin.com

Contents

THE NEW
NATIONAL
HEALTH
SERVICE

*

Your new National Health Service begins on 5th July. What is it? How do you get it?

It will provide you with all medical, dental, and nursing care. Everyone—rich or poor, man, woman or child—can use it or any part of it. There are no charges, except for a few special items. There are no insurance qualifications. But it is not a "charity". You are all paying for it, mainly as taxpayers, and it will relieve your money worries in time of illness.

'Medical treatment should be made available to rich and poor alike in accordance with medical need and no other criteria. Worry about money in a time of sickness is a serious hindrance to recovery, apart from its unnecessary cruelty. The essence of a satisfactory health service is that the rich and poor are treated alike. Poverty is not a disability and wealth is not an advantage.'

Aneurin Bevan, 1946 speech to the House of Commons

Introduction

The State of Medicine

I am furious sad, and scared for the NHS. Like many – most – doctors, I wondered how not to be a cliché at my interview for medical school. How to say that I felt I had a vocation, that I wanted to do something useful and of value to others without sounding trite? Yet I did, and I – even more old-fashionedly – love my job. I adore it. The pleasure of being a useful part of people's lives is not just intellectually satisfying but fulfilling on a deep, human level. Working in medicine, in the National Health Service, is the best job in the world. Our NHS is a phenomenal achievement. For NHS natives like me, having grown up with it – and now practising medicine in Scotland, which is protected from the worst of the Health and Social Care Act – it would be easy to think that the NHS will always be with us. It won't, unless we collectively want it enough to make sure it is.

I write as Jeremy Hunt, the longest-serving Secretary of State for Health to date, is set to impose a new junior doctors' contract. I loved and hated being a junior doctor in equal measure. The hours then, as now, are long, and the responsibilities overwhelming. I only got through the year because of the unending support of my colleagues – from the consultant who realised I was knackered after 48 hours on call and took my pager off me, ordering me home to sleep, to the other juniors who unfailingly stayed late and helped out when there were more patients than time (often). This sort of goodwill – driven by vocation and fuelled by kindness – cannot be bought and sold. It can be lost, through tiredness, resentment, hurt, anger and despair. It can be flushed away when people feel badly treated and when the joy that keeps many professionals going – the feeling that one is doing a good job, a useful job – evaporates. The moral contract between professionals and patients is more important than any financial one. Threatening the goodwill – which is cement to the bricks of the NHS – as Hunt did when he implied that juniors did not already work at weekends, or were no longer professionals, makes morale crumble. Along with clinical competence and adequate resources, staff morale is vital because without it we lose that goodwill, both the cement and the rocket fuel of NHS organisation.

For medicine is a vocation, that old-fashioned thing. It is not commerce. Over the last few years, commercial relationships have been dripped into the NHS, with accompanying advertising, competition and evaluations, surrounded by an entourage of management consultants, led by politicians spinning the evidence, publicised by soundbites and popularity contests. Looking on from Scotland, I am aghast. Cuts to the NHS have been savage – a £20 billion savings target was in place in 2015,[1] with an extra £1.5 billion to be saved in 2016 – but the austerity budget has also been placed across social care and public health. The NHS constitution is a calm reminder of what the service is meant to stand for. Yet the strain it is now under is immense and cannot be sustained indefinitely. GP surgeries are closing, NHS Trusts are running out of money, private providers are relinquishing contracts part-way through a term and junior doctors are leaving for Australia. Slow motion crumble doesn't attract as much attention as an almighty sudden crash.

Is this then a fait accompli? Should the NHS be declared unfit for modern purpose and allowed to die? Absolutely not. This book examines the evidence for what we are doing to our NHS. It is the best hope we have for fairly distributing healthcare. While the constitution of the NHS should be timeless, the underlying philosophy of how we decide what the NHS spends its resources on requires fundamental rethinking. Simply, we need to stop doing things that don't work. We repeatedly start the NHS off on short-term, poorly thought out and highly politicised cul-de-sacs that are later evaluated – once the money has run out – only to find much waste and little benefit for patients. Frankly, we should forbid any new policy without knowing what the harms – for there are always harms – will be. We should not spend more money than we have to. We can stop doing things of no or low value. We should not base what the NHS does on party politics, but long-term appreciation of the evidence, the benefits and the risks.

At the start, the NHS provided basic care to a population that had known very little. Now it is creating bespoke treatments for people with particular genetically driven cancers, offering renal dialysis to people in their 80s and 90s and performing heart transplants – a dream far distant from Bevan's proposals. Dying patients can have daily, or more, visits from the GP or district nurse in order to have quality terminal care at home. Opportunities for spending on high-tech healthcare can gallop in front of any reasonable budget. The advent of NICE, the National Institute for Clinical Excellence (now the National Institute for Health and Care Excellence), in 1999 was an attempt to formally search for 'value for money' on drugs or operations, but it has endured much criticism as well as political attempts to thwart it. NICE has been bypassed, as have other organisations such as the National Screening Committee, by numerous political policies, introduced without any attempts to seek critical appraisal or act on it. This is full-frontal daylight robbery and if we want the NHS to exist, it cannot continue.

The NHS is more than science or evidence, and the evidence itself may not always be clear, be disputed or be uncertain. The constitution of the NHS is enacted by an interwoven tangle of human beings. This week, I listened extra carefully to media coverage of the NHS, and have not spotted any headline or proposal that takes into account any supposition that staff may already be doing their best. So, care for strokes was *failing* and care for the dying *must improve*.

The motivations of staff were implicitly assumed to be poor and careless. Yet so much of human care and kindness rests on the motivations of the people who work and use the NHS. Policymaking frequently sidesteps or belittles the enormous resource of the people whose life story is also an NHS story. This is why each chapter of this book is preceded by interviews with people who have important insights into the NHS or healthcare delivery more broadly: a nurse who trained in the 1950s, a doctor who worked at Mid Staffs, a US economist and a patient with a terminal illness. Each illuminates the strengths, ethos of and challenges faced by the NHS. The NHS is not just a story of statistics and spending; it is a story of belonging, loyalty, vocation, life, pride, passion and joy. But how often are professionals and patients in the NHS seen as a source of information and advice to policymakers? How many are seen as irritations in the way of the change that is being levered in, rather than assistants in knowing what is needed and what is not? So when a nurse tells us of the pleasure in wearing her uniform half a century ago, or a doctor describes how – despite doing nothing wrong and everything to help – a legal investigation profoundly affected him, or how a patient facing terminal illness feels reassured by the relationship they have with their doctor, I hope that the shared values of the NHS shine with enough resonance that we stop to consider: are we willing to assemble ourselves with the necessary vigour to defend the NHS from being stripped of goodwill and morally devalued?

Interview

Belinda Hull, *retired nurse and midwife*

The first of January 1958 was the day that changed my life forever when I entered nurse training at the Ipswich and East Suffolk Hospital, Anglesea Road Wing.

I had left school aged 15 and for the previous three years had been an office junior. A fill-in job until I was old enough to start nurse training at 18.

The first three months of training were spent in PTS, Preliminary Training School. We were not permitted to wear our caps until we started ward work. We were issued with three dresses, three caps, six collars and 14 aprons, all of which were starched to the stiffness of cardboard by the laundry each week. Our dresses were a lovely shade of lilac but at the end of three and a half years you were happy to exchange them for the pale blue of a Staff Nurse, plus of course a frilly cap. Student caps were plain and held on with white hairgrips. We were also issued with a warm woolly nurse's cape, navy on the outside, lined with red, which we wore inside out at Christmas when we sang carols around the wards – an impressive sight.

My first ward was male surgical, Felix Ward, commanded by Sister Larter. A formidable, strict, workaholic whose life revolved around Felix. She was strict, fair, a stickler for efficiency: the bed wheels all had to point the same way around for consultants' rounds, which were conducted rather like the queen inspecting a guard of honour. Felix was Sister Larter.

I think that all the sisters were held in enormously high regard by the consultants. The respect went both ways. All the sisters lived in the Sisters' Home, Oaklands, and all the nurses lived in the Nurses' Home, Norton House. The sisters seemed to see their work as their calling in life, rather like a nun. At Anglesea Road we had 25 ward/departmental sisters of whom only one was married and lived off site. They lived in hospital accommodation until retirement.

We were held in very high esteem by the public. We were recognised and respected, offered seats on a crowded bus or train. We were also given free tickets for the theatre and dances organised at the local army, air force and naval bases.

In PTS we learned and practised basic nursing care before being let loose on the wards. We had lectures on anatomy, physiology, health and hygiene, lifting and handling, and practised bedmaking, bed baths, care of patients' hair, nails and teeth, and care of pressure areas. We spent a lot of time learning how to bandage every part of the body with cotton bandages, which were endlessly rewound on a special handheld winding machine. The mainstay of pressure area care revolved around the 'back round', which was carried out on every bedbound patient in the hospital usually four-hourly but more frequently if sister deemed it necessary. We did the theory in the classroom before we put it into practice on the ward.

In 1959 I remember Miss Gooch, sister tutor, saying to us: 'Mark my words girls. The injudicious use of antibiotics will be the death of us.' The early days of my nursing career predated intensive care units. Seriously ill or injured patients were 'specialled' on medical and surgical wards by one nurse, not part of the ward team. These nurses had no extra training for the role and we had limited resources with which to treat patients. Many of these patients did not survive. Intensive Therapy Units (ITUs) were set up soon after this.

Our first year of ward work revolved around basic nursing care, an endless round of washing patients, caring for pressure areas, making beds and feeding and hydrating patients. A lot of time was spent filling in fluid balance charts and ensuring that patients had sufficient intake of fluids to meet their needs. Fluid balance is all fluids in (for example, drink, naso-gastric tube) set against all fluids out (urine, drainage bottles, wound drainage). This was critical to the wellbeing of the patients on a surgical ward who had recently undergone surgery for gastric/duodenal ulcers, a common procedure then. As patients improved they were moved into the wing before going to a convalescent home for further recovery/rehabilitation before returning home. No such luxury today, even though recovery from an operation causing the same trauma still takes the same amount of time as then. Patients just expect to get better quicker.

All nurses were involved at mealtimes assisting patients who were unable to feed themselves. This was a nursing task and the nutrition of each patient was overseen by sister, who served the food. Sister knew everything about every patient and therefore planned all their care. In succeeding years this became known as 'the nursing process' and was devolved down to all nurses caring for a small group of patients. During my early nursing years we were very task-orientated (we carried out a specific task for all patients and then did a different task for all patients). 'The nursing process', which involved nurses carrying out all tasks for one patient before moving to the next patient, put paid to that – but it was a very efficient method of delivering care to all patients. The nursing process reduces the number of times a patient is disturbed but also reduces the time when a nurse is interacting with a patient.

The patients had their evening cocoa, Ovaltine or Horlicks when we started our night shift and were settled for the night by about 10 p.m. After 10 p.m. the wards went quiet. We recognised that sleep was important for sick patients and that sleep is usually easier if it is quiet. Nurses and doctors communicated in hushed tones and shoes were silent. Throughout the night we would sit at a long table making swabs and dressing packs to pack into metal drums, which were sent to be sterilised in the hospital autoclave next morning, collected and delivered by the porters.

Collecting specimens of urine was an occupational hazard. Sluices were full of them and the smell was awful. Every day sister had to compile a list of patients who were dangerously ill (the DIL), which was sent to matron. Matron would appear on the ward most days and be taken around by sister.

In 1958 I remember a big party at Heath Road to celebrate the first ten years of the NHS. Whatever consultants, other doctors and nurses thought about the NHS before it was formed, I was not aware that anyone did not wholeheartedly approve of it ten years later.

By today's standards theatres were prehistoric. Instruments were stored in glass cabinets and were hand-selected by qualified staff for procedures identified from the operating list. Weekends were taken up by emptying, cleaning and restocking glass dishes and jars containing blades, needles and suture material; which were sterilised in Ethicon fluid or Lysol – a powerful fluid which could burn your skin. Another mammoth task was the washing, drying and turning, powdering and repacking of surgeons' gloves. There were so many linen lines in the pack room with dozens of rubber gloves drying before checking for holes and packing in drums for sterilising. The drums had holes around the side, which were open during steam sterilisation and were closed after drying by porters. Washing surgeons' used gloves was an unpleasant task. Another task favoured by sisters was to upend all the trolleys, remove, clean and replace the wheels – they tended to get sutures wrapped around the wheels, which stopped them running freely.

Used swabs were counted and discarded into a bucket and then had to be hung up on a swab rack, using Cheatle forceps, by the circulating nurse, who most frequently was a student. They were then counted again at the end of every procedure.

At this time, 1959, children could be diagnosed with phenylketonuria (PK), and could only be treated with special diets. These children were admitted to hospital and needed a diet which did not contain phenylalanine. It was during this time that treatment became available and all babies were tested for PK soon after birth. This transformed the lives of affected children who otherwise failed to develop normally, leading to learning difficulties. Their bodies were unable to metabolise phenylalanine.

After six months as a staff nurse on women's surgical, I embarked on midwifery training. I was six months shadowing a qualified midwife on home visits on a bicycle. I was fortunate enough to deliver 29 babies in the six-month period. Most low-risk women were delivered of their babies in their own home. The mantra was 'the best place to have a baby is at home' because emergencies could (in theory if not always in practice) be dealt with by the 'Flying Squad'. Home meant less risk of infection, there was a continuity of midwife care and the women were generally more relaxed in their own home. This has now almost gone full circle.

I went back to theatres. I soon requested a transfer and was offered a junior sister role in ophthalmics, where I learned and grew in a happy environment. We ran a small ward, outpatients and our own theatre list. One of the happiest times in my 49-year career – I understood the anatomy well and enjoyed the slow, quiet, gentle, meticulous way of working, which suited me. One had to be slow and quiet, because most of the patients could not see and one had to be careful not to startle them.

In the early 60s we did not wear surgical gloves. They were not sensitive enough for eye surgeons to use. Most of the work we did was removing cataracts under local anaesthesia, but unlike today the patients were in hospital on bed rest for a week post-operatively. This was known as 'bed absolute care'. These patients were heavily sedated to discourage them from too much movement.

I retired from nursing in 2007, after 47 years of service, finishing in NHS Direct. NHS Direct was an excellent service but sadly too costly to maintain with trained nurses. I wouldn't have missed my career in the NHS for the world.

1

The Promise of the NHS

At midnight on 4 July 1948 the National Health Service was born. Aneurin Bevan – Welsh, socialist, radical, passionate – was the health secretary who made himself the NHS's midwife. Britain was at the end of two world wars, its population of young men withered, its people still using food coupons – one egg, 8 oz of butter and 8 oz of cheese a week. Tuberculosis, whooping cough, tetanus and diphtheria were the regular killers of children.[1] The average life expectancy of a man born then was less than 60.[2] Scarce cars, no internet, few households had telephones, baths were had twice a week and outside toilets were normal. It was a different world. Healthcare had been provided by a mixture of (limited) charity and direct payments to hospitals and general practitioners. No money: no doctor.

Bevan recognised that the stress and worry caused by paying for healthcare was harmful. He said: *'To millions of people below the "salaried job" level security is almost as tangible a thing as money itself; to know that bad luck will not mean acute poverty is to be free of the most persistent and stabbing anxiety which afflicts the wage-earner.'*

He went on: *'The whole population becomes, for the first time, entitled to the medical services hitherto available only to insured workers; the scandal of "under-doctored" areas will slowly disappear. But the full fruit of these reforms will not be ripe until the system of health centres has had time to grow, and that growth would be gradual even if lack of bricks and mortar did not inhibit it at the start. One must think of the health service as a huge natural organism in process of growth, not as a creature of magic, called out of the void by the wand of the Minister of Health.'* [3]

Yet, as I will explain, the NHS continues to be expected to operate as a *'creature of magic'* by its political masters. We have failed to get beyond party politics and the continual creation of bad policies which have wasted money, time and effort – and which have resulted in less quality and quantity of life for people and their families than is possible.

Bevan, in campaigning relentlessly for the NHS, was famously opposed – not just by Conservatives and members of his own Labour Party, but by doctors, chiefly in the form of the British Medical Association (BMA) (which then as now represents the vast majority of doctors in the UK). The BMA's secretary Dr Charles Hill – already well known for his national radio topics on medical issues – campaigned ardently against the formation of the NHS. Remarkably, the debates which he was having 70 years ago are contemporarily prescient. How much have we really moved on? During a BBC radio interview between Hill and a surgeon, Bourne, arguing against him in 1943, Hill said:

'In my view the services of this country are good. They are continually improving. I admit they lack co-ordination, and that they overlap and have certain disadvantages. In my view, all these can easily be organised by organisation. I see no reason whatever to bring doctors into the position of the civil service as full-time officers.'

His opponent, meantime, was unimpressed: *'But all those who speak from your point of view speak with this bogey of the civil service. You have in your mind that medical services which are organised for the state, will be on the same level of routine and unimaginative conduct as some branches of the present civil service. But that's an assumption which isn't justified.'*

Hill responded, *'Well then, let's thrash this out. There's a feeling, quite widespread, that to some extent, based on experience in this war, what's called the "cold hand of bureaucratic control", that it does descend on a service that is administered by the state.'*

What's missing in the discussion is something vital – evidence about what level of bureaucracy is necessary, and whether 'routine', standard care is a good or bad thing. Bourne confronts Hill with the evidence of a local hospital that had been taken into 'guardianship', or state control:

'They've improved out of all recognition. The more advanced of them now compete for efficiency and progress with any of the voluntary hospitals. Where does the dead hand of bureaucracy come in there? These public-controlled hospitals are encouraged to be the growing points of medicine.'

The very same wrestling with whether state versus private control of hospitals is good or bad repeats itself today. The multinational company Circle had a private contract to run Hinchingbrooke Hospital between 2010 and 2015, and many people questioned the wisdom of this relinquishing of state control to the private sector. In the 1943 debate Hill challenged public service on the grounds of inefficiency. Bourne countered, arguing that doctors should be civil servants, a point that is just as relevant today. He said:

'I believe that medicine should not be regarded by those who enter the profession as a means of making money in the ordinary sense of the phrase. A salary, pension, holidays, and postgraduate facilities with reduced expenses of upkeep and establishment would attract the right type of man or women to medicine, which is really vocational and not a business or trade.'

Hill was unconvinced, replying: *'You believe that competition between doctors is undesirable? You don't agree that it's a necessary stimulus to individual good work?'*

'I don't agree that it is a necessary stimulus. I think it brings out some of the worst features in medical practice. Such as competition for patients, unnecessary fancy visiting of the rich, attempts to take patients from each other, and currying favour with the patient by the means of parting from the medical necessities of the case?'

Hill challenged him: *'And you don't think that the effort of a doctor to obtain a bigger practice and more patients is an incitement to work well, to work better?'*

'No, it's an incitement to a bigger income.'

'Better work?'

'Not necessarily, because the better quality of work can't be measured by the fees paid.'

'But it is measured by the fees paid! The doctor who does bad work soon loses his practice!'

'By no means, the patient on the whole is unable to judge the quality of the doctor's work.'

'Then who is able to judge? In my view the patient is as well able to judge as anybody. There is no body or committee which is any more likely to choose a good doctor than the patient themselves.'

'A patient's judgement as to whether a doctor is good is largely based on pleasant social manners. The bedside manner, so-called, his ability to make himself pleasing to the family and to prescribe such treatments as the patient may feel he should have.'

This argument could just as easily have been had this year. From the 2010s, the political ideology was to encourage competition and comparisons between local GP practices, with patients encouraged to rate and compare local services and change doctors if they wished. The Conservative and Liberal Democrat coalition government between 2010 and 2015 promoted such competition using phraseology such as 'patient choice', and by means of internet rating sites for doctors it trusted in the premise that patients know good services when they see them, will report their opinions, such that other potential patients will change doctor to a well-rated one, and that this competition will drive up standards.

To this argument, Bourne remained unconvinced: 'By all means let's have a pleasing bedside manner – let it be an incidental – but a doctor who is imperfectly equipped as a doctor can now make up for that lack by having a pleasant manner and pandering to his patients wants and tastes.'

This is exactly the fear that doctors in this decade have expressed about the push to popularity ratings, a concept that will be explored in detail later. It is telling that the same ideas and counter-arguments are parried over a distance of 70 years. Hill was arguing that patients must be free to choose a doctor; Bourne that free choice is already, in a private system, skewed, and unlikely to happen in any case.

Workload was one of the few subjects the men agreed on: *'There must be many fewer patients to each doctor. Whereas, right now, a doctor may have up to 2,500 on his panel.'*

'Yes, the average is about a thousand.'

'He shouldn't have more than a thousand, and the present elaboration of diagnostic and treatment measures, it's certain that he'd do better work if he had many fewer, because he'd have more time for each patient.'

'Then you'd want a multiplication of the medical profession before you can cope with the reforms?'

'Yes, there must be many more doctors ... Nothing must stand between the doctor and patient.'[4]

The average list size of a general practitioner in the UK in 2012 was just under 1,600 people.[5] This is a rise since 1948, despite the instinct one might have to require more GPs. After all, we live longer lives and there has been a colossal shift of work from hospitals into general practice. In the 1980s it was common for most people with type 2 diabetes to be seen in hospital outpatients regularly, as were people with high blood pressure. Now this is the exception, not the rule. Minor surgery, fitting long-term contraception, treating and regularly reviewing the millions of people who have chronic diseases like bronchitis and diabetes, long-term care for people who have had a stroke, or who have depression: this work is now done in primary care, mainly by GPs, with practice nurses and sometimes pharmacists to assist. In 1948 the complaint was that there were not enough GPs; in 2014, the Royal College of GPs launched a campaign saying exactly the same thing.

Similarly, one of Bourne's sentiments – *'I don't believe that a doctor needs a financial incentive to do good work'*, as he put it – is identically argued in the 21st century. General practitioners are not, in the main, direct employees of the NHS, but are contracted to the NHS. As a GP, I am paid according to how many patients I have on the practice list – about £136 per year per patient.[6] The practice staff – nurses, receptionists, managers, cleaners – are paid for by the GPs and out of the total funding, which comes from the NHS. In practice this means that to ensure stability, GPs have to take on most or all of the 'enhanced services' or 'incentive' payments for vaccinations and screening. In 2015, GP Gavin Francis wrote that:

The government's health policy reached new levels of absurdity last October, when it was announced that GPs would be paid £55 for every diagnosis of dementia they could enter in a patient's notes. It was to be a short-term initiative, set to expire before May's general election – it's said the Department of Health was keen to meet a target.[7]

This conflict between trusting doctors to do the professional and 'right thing' regardless of financial incentives (as Bourne implied) versus promoting competition for patients and financial rewards to make staff act in particular ways has not been resolved over almost 70 years. Some of this might be because they are moral principles based on a belief system. Providing incentives and engendering competition tends to reflect the views, broadly, of the political right while the principle of providing equal services appeals more to the political left. But there is another way forward.

Left and Right are united in an overwhelming consensus (at least publicly) to revere the NHS. Prior to the 2015 general election, David Cameron urged citizens[8] to trust him on the future of the NHS: *'I can guarantee you today: we will not endanger universal coverage – we will make sure it remains a National Health Service. ... We will not break up or hinder efficient and integrated care – we will improve it.'*[9] So, too, agreed Norman Lamb, Minister of State for Care and Support: *'Our NHS is our most treasured public service and it is safe in Liberal Democrat hands,'* he said prior to the 2015 general election.[10] Shona Robinson, of the Scottish Nationalist Party, described the NHS as *'our most cherished public service.'*[11]

Or Ed Miliband, previous Labour leader, who said: *'I don't need to tell you here that the NHS is the most precious* institution in our country. We all have our own reasons why we love the NHS. It looks after us when we're born. It cares for us when we're sick. And it so often cares for us also in our final days and weeks of life. It is the proudest achievement in our country and the envy of the world.'[12]

The main political parties thus agree that the NHS is an iconic ideal, profound in its effects, and that they wish to support and cherish it. To this end, Bevan's construct stands firm – at least in terms of expressed contemporary political belief. However, Bevan's Fabian Lecture of 1950 is instructive. After reminding us that democracy has only been won in the last 25 years, and that many countries have not obtained it, he talks about unemployment and tells us of the housewife:

'... she knows very well at the end of the week that if she has so much money and it all goes, and she wants to do something more, if she wants to buy an extra pair of shoes or send a child to the cinema twice instead of once – God help him! – then she has to do it at the expense of some other member of the family, some other form of expenditure. She must exercise, in her own domain, this principle of selection; but no one seems to have recognised that the same principle applies to society, applies to the national economy. It carries extraordinary implications, and you have it before your very eyes.'

Bevan also asks, if everyone is in full employment 'and we want to do something more than we are doing, at whose expense is it going to be done?' What would we put first in the national order of things? He appealed for a citizenry that was capable of determining who goes to the head of the queue and who goes to the bottom of the queue, a civilised position that created a hierarchical order of values, some above the others: 'So you are reaching a new kind of authoritarian society, but it is the authority of a moral purpose freely undertaken.'[13]

As Bevan spoke these words, it is unlikely that he would have been imagining the scenario where the NHS would be asked to fund drug treatment costing upwards of one-third of a million pounds per year.[14] It is unlikely that he would have been imagining that contracts for the care of older people would be sold to the lowest bidder.[15] I cannot imagine Bevan standing before his audience, explaining the need for society to share moral judgements on how money should be spent, while also imagining that one day the chief executives of hospitals, charged with performance targets, would be paid ten or more times that of nurses.[16]

Bevan's insight recognises that resources are finite, that distributing resources is a duty, and caring for our sick is a duty society should share. He is asking citizens and patients to take responsibility for deciding who should get attention and resources last – that they and not just doctors had to make these choices. Bourne, arguing with Hill, was saying that there should be an organisational level between the state and the doctor, with *'wide representation of the profession as well as of the patient'* – a statement with which Hill agreed. This may have taken 70 years, but it has turned out to be only partly enacted in the form of organisations like the National Institute for Health and Care Excellence (NICE), the Scottish Medicines Consortium or the National Screening Committee (NSC). It is telling that at the inception of the NHS, both the limits on resources and the need for citizens and patients to be involved in organising and distributing them were recognised. These dilemmas and tensions still exist. But our politicians are united in stating that they adhere to the principles of the universality of the NHS. If so, there is a non-party political way that can be steered through these tensions: what works for patients? What is best to spend our money on? What way of working – incentives or professional contracts – gives the best care for people?

Why should we be bothered about any of this? June Hautot has written 'I was born outside it, so I know how difficult it is to live without it. I saw my father going to work when he was very ill, because he couldn't afford to take time off. My mother was ill and he had to pay five shillings for the doctor, our rent was only 12 shillings, so he had to work even though he had emphysema. In those days you couldn't afford to be ill – and that's what's going to happen again.'[17]

The NHS is not *'magic'*. It has been called into being through a collective conviction, hard work, grit and the humanity of its workers, who every day do a little bit more than they are paid to do, who stay late, who arrive early, who skip lunch, who take the extra moment to speak to a relative rather than catching the next bus home. The NHS was always going to be an organisation making hard choices on finite resources; however, it is now dissolving at the edges, dipped into the worlds of Private Finance Initiatives (PFIs), corroded through GP contracts and pummelled by political demands whose unrealism only take away that finite resource directly from patients.

Two or three generations have been born, lived and died in the NHS. Its constant presence – like cars, mobile phones and wifi – has meant a population of people who have grown up as NHS natives. But the NHS is not a given; it only continues to exist because we will it and want it to be so. I will show how the NHS is repeating errors in policy and practice that could be avoided, and that it is being bent to short-term populist political appeal rather than aspiring to moral and humane practice. The tragedy is that this slow erosion may not be noticed widely enough – never mind protested against – until the NHS has become a carcass, devoured by commercial and political self-interest. This book is both a review of the state of the art of medicine and a plea that we wake up to what is happening to our NHS and demand that our politicians love it like they say they do.

Chris Turner, consultant in A&E

I'd worked in lots of different places: I thought I knew what good looked like. And then I went to Mid Staffs. Going in the doors it was obvious that something was wrong.

The emergency department seemed to float differently from the rest of the hospital. It was a 'bastard child' – in a bad sense. The organisation threatened junior nurses with the sack if they allowed breaches (in targets) – if you are a band 5 nurse [junior nurse] you maybe don't know that you can't be sacked for making that happen. The sole driver was the financial pressure the hospital was under. Breaches were nothing to do with quality of care – I never heard anyone talking about quality of care, until the Healthcare Commission came along. I don't think it was a deliberate omission on the part of the management guys. They were solely focused on the money. They got themselves into a position where they couldn't hear what everyone else was saying about the quality of care. They became deaf and blind to the quality of care. It was all about money. Within the nursing hierarchy there were senior people who believed you could provide very good quality of care by using a very unusual model of nurses – basically bunching them across the hospital, saying they could slot into one job or another because they have a 'generic set of competencies'. But you can't quantify the gestalt that nurses get over the years. It's like saying that no doctors are ever specialists. So when a nurse asks you to see a patient 'now' – and they are right to because they know the patient is sick – it's not a sixth sense, it's experiential sense. At Mid Staffordshire Trust they were going for the lowest common denominator of nursing care – actually below that. The experience of nurses [in the wards] wasn't respected at all.

I'd gone up the chain, as you're meant to do. I'd even spoken to the chief executive. I had been one of the people who went to the Healthcare Commission and said: 'It's not good what's happening here.' I felt as though I was speaking a different language to everyone else. The problem was all financial. Quality of care had no place. Management was all about making it cheaper and cheaper and cheaper to provide healthcare. Clinicians who felt marginalised had stopped engaging with management. One consultant – who is no longer practising – was very disruptive. His frustration at the organisation came out in a very unhelpful way.

I wasn't prepared, on a personal level, to compromise what I wanted to be as a doctor and fit into that culture. I wasn't alone in Mid Staffs, there were lots of other people who wanted to provide good care. We slowly started to change it, and it got quicker once the Healthcare Commission got involved. There had been a lot of hostility from other departments to the emergency department [ED] – such as 'let the real doctors look after patients'. The prevailing atmosphere was that the ED was a bad place – they weren't wrong. The department was effectively dislocated from the rest of the hospital. We were trying to change it.

At first I didn't feel that I was allowed to care. But my colleagues and I got absorbed into it, trying to fix it. We were putting in 80-hour weeks, plus on call on top. I had no problem with doing that. We started to support junior doctors and junior nurses; we provided a degree of shielding from the other stuff that was coming down from the organisation by involving ourselves in conversations with the senior (management) guys – rather than saying, 'bugger off, we were doing our best'. It seemed to make a difference: retention was better, our staff appeared happier, our mortality rate was down, and I was genuinely proud to work there. I was proud of the difference we'd made. As time went by, I began to learn that the staff were working beyond the limit at which they could manage to do all the niceties and their job.

Once the Francis Report came out, we (in the department) were in a different world. We were then in a department that cared about safety, we were explicit about what it meant to work there – we want to do our best, treat patients in a way that's acceptable for our families, and when we are not, we will look at it, and try and do something about it, if we can. So we talked about the experience that patients had as they were in the department and provided education for all members of the department. Up till then, education had just been shoved to the side because there wasn't time to do it. There had also been times in the past that training was cancelled because there had been too many breaches (of the four-hour target) the previous day. It was punitive. The idea of getting people in a room together isn't just about learning how to treat something, it's also about understanding behaviours and being open and clear – what it meant to be a doctor, what it meant to be a nurse. That education hadn't been valued before.

Patients were scared. The newspapers were saying that we were the hospital of death, that we had a one and a half times the national average death rate. Actually, by this point our HSMR [Hospital Standardised Mortality Ratio] was running at 60% of the national average and we were probably providing as good care as anyone in the UK at that point. We still made mistakes. Our mistakes were under the magnifying glass. Patients were naturally extremely anxious about coming in. Some of them were openly hostile. It was very difficult to deal with. One of the nurses was told by a patient that she was no better than 'shit on my shoe'.

When good people do unacceptable things in the NHS it is rarely – in fact I would say never – inexcusable. So the nurse leaves three patients who have soiled themselves in a bed – that's all you hear. But the rest of the story is that there was one nurse for 24 patients – and one of them was dying. And that nurse spent her time trying to sort out what needed to happen for that person. Yes, that is unacceptable, it is however not inexcusable for that nurse – it's understandable; it is, though, unacceptable and inexcusable on a corporate level.

I carry a very personal guilt. When the nurses went to the NMC [National Medical Council] (for disciplinary hearings) I should have been there to give that clinical perspective and explain what was happening in the hospital at that time. But at the time I was broken, I was completely broken. I wasn't able to deal with this at that point. When they got struck off I think they were, to a certain extent, scapegoated.

2

In Need of Care –
the State of the Modern NHS

Does the NHS deserve to be cherished? It is the issue people are most likely to consider when voting.[1] Yet the NHS has failed abysmally, and many times: Mid Staffs, Shipman, Bristol children's heart surgery, Morecambe Bay – these were scandals when the NHS did not just *let people down* but actively killed, harmed or maimed. These have caused massive, avoidable suffering for both patients and staff. They have been followed by public inquiries, apologies and promises that such things should never happen again. But the environment in which such catastrophes were allowed to happen has not changed in ways that would give consistent high-quality care the best possible chance. Instead, the NHS lacks mandatory safe staffing and remains stuffed with targets, which can end up doing more harm than good. The question should no longer be *'will we ever learn?'* but *'how do we build the NHS to ensure that we don't have to learn the same lesson ever again?'*

The shame of Mid Staffs

The public inquiry chaired by Robert Francis QC was set up in the wake of an investigation by the Healthcare Commission (the forerunner to the Care Quality Commission, or CQC) into Mid Staffordshire NHS Foundation Trust in 2009, because the hospital had high mortality rates, and the inquiry report was published in 2013.[2]

The investigation had found multiple, awful problems. The quality of information being gathered at Mid Staffs about surgery or Accident and Emergency (A&E) attendances was poor. There weren't enough doctors or nurses. The nurses hadn't been given the right training to use equipment, such as heart monitors. There were delays of days for emergency surgery for people who had broken their hip – leading to patients being 'nil by mouth' and not given the medication they needed. There weren't enough beds, with chronic staff shortages. Junior doctors were given too much responsibility. Oversight was lacking. In October 2007, a patient went missing from a ward and was found dead half a mile away five days later. Although a discussion about what happened occurred in February 2008, an investigation into it did not occur until almost a year afterwards. What the management team thought was happening was entirely different from what was actually happening. Relatives told the inquiry how family members had been denied food, water or access to the toilet, were not washed properly or were in pain but ignored.

The Healthcare Commission published its report in 2009. In 2006/7 the hospital Trust had a target to save £10 million, planning a surplus of £1 million. To achieve this surplus the trust sacked 150 staff and took away 18% of beds (over 100 in total). The CQC reported that *'in 2005, the Trust had more wards with below the national average number of nurses than wards with above the average, by almost two to one'*, and it found *'a shortfall of 120 whole time equivalent nursing posts'*. The result was a hospital stripped down to the bones. One doctor later said in his statement to Francis: *'I would often see two nurses run ragged doing what six should have been doing ... If one of those nurses went off sick there would be only one left. If there had been more nurses, none of this would have happened.'*

Another doctor recalled that *'an old man on ward 11 pressed a buzzer over and over again as he wanted to urinate. He was a frail chap with poor mobility, and as the buzzer was not answered, he eventually went to the loo in the early hours of the morning and broke a hip. He went for surgery and died the next day.'*

Staff shortages were not limited to nurses. A doctor said that because of a *'virtual collapse of administrative support'*

> 'It was quite normal for nurses to come out at the end of these meetings crying because they had been told that if they did not meet the four-hour targets, they would lose their jobs. This sometimes happened several times in a week. Had there been a matron-like figure ... the situation might well have been different, but there was no one sufficiently senior to correct this misinformation and intimidation which the nurses were receiving from middle management at this time.'[3]

the results of scans showing cancer were not given to him for months afterwards. He added that the lack of nurses meant that they did not regularly attend consultant ward rounds, which *'constitutes a serious clinical risk issue and has the potential of undermining patient care'*. Nurses on ward rounds typically report on how the patient is doing, sharing information and helping to plan discharge with the doctor, although the rounds also take a nurse away from direct patient care on the ward.

One nurse told Francis that many newly recruited nurses were very junior, with *'no experience and were terrified at the level of work they had to do'*. She went on:

'Nurses were expected to break the rules as a matter of course in order to meet targets, a prime example of this being the maximum four-hour wait time target for patients in A&E. Rather than "breach" the target, the length of waiting time would regularly be falsified on notes and computer records.'

The nurse described how managing other nurses placed her under pressure to lie in the records, having been told that if they didn't meet the targets, heads would roll and A&E would be closed, with everyone losing their jobs: *'I understood this point but I was equally concerned about the terrible effect that our actions were having on patient care.'* Well-intentioned targets meant that hospitals had to either discharge or admit people attending A&E within four hours, or the hospital was fined. She had to fill in reports about why patients had not been discharged before the four-hour target was up: *'I was up till 1 a.m. typing my report, even though I was back on shift at 7 a.m.'* As for the targets themselves: *'It is a good idea to have targets,'* she said, *'but the system is being completely abused. Patients are still lying on trolleys for 12 hours, they are just doing it in a different room; a room which is not classed as A&E.'*

The four-hour target and A&E pressures

The four-hour target was introduced by Labour after it won the general election in 1997. A&E is a front door to the NHS. There are no limits on how many people can attend on a single day. It is a rare event for a hospital to declare itself overwhelmed and to divert ambulances to another hospital – in general, staff just have to deal with whoever needs them. Like primary care, staff in A&E have to see as many people who have, or are believed to have, a need for care. It is an open door into a room without a ceiling.

In 1992, 13 million people went to A&E for treatment; by 1999 it was 14.6 million[4] and in 2012 it was 18.3 million.[5] As a result of this rising demand, people were waiting in A&E for unacceptably long times for many treatments – for example, an 84-year-old man waited for more than 28 hours in A&E before he was taken to a ward. In response to this demand, the government's plan for the NHS made it clear that there needed to be greater investment. More doctors were employed and nurses were trained to look after patients with minor complaints from door to discharge home. In 2002, 23% of patients waited four hours or more in A&E; by 2007, 97.7% of patients were assessed, treated and discharged in four hours.

Superficially, the target looks like a major success story, yet the evidence of the A&E nurse from Mid Staffs is disturbing. The then Mid Staffs NHS Trust was in the process of trying to become a Foundation Trust (FT), a status being offered to hospitals if they had achieved certain ratings from the Healthcare Commission and one that would[6] allow them more financial autonomy, to be able to keep the proceeds of land sales, and freed from being directly 'line managed' by the central NHS.[7] But just as Mid Staffs aspired to meet the criteria for FT status, it was losing a lot of nurses.

Until 2004, hospitals were under the control of government and managed by local health authorities. Alan Milburn, the then Labour health secretary, instigated a new 'Foundation Trust' (FT) status for hospitals. To be allowed FT status, hospitals were to meet certain criteria and be approved by the independent evaluator, Monitor. Hospitals with FT status are self-standing, self-governing and 'free to determine their own future'.[8] They manage their own surplus money, choosing how and when to borrow and what to spend it on. Foundation Trusts have a duty to consult and involve a board of governors who include patients, staff, citizens and 'partner organisations'. Government policy was for all hospitals to become FTs by 2014.[9] Wales and Northern Ireland do not have Foundation Trusts.

The official reaction to the Francis inquiry

The government made a long response to the Francis inquiry. It proposed new safety schemes, such as quarterly safety reports, a new patient safety programme and monthly publication of ward-by-ward staffing levels. It also said it would minimise bureaucracy in order to free time for staff to care for patients, instruct hospitals to put the name of the responsible nurse and consultant above each patient's bed, and create a 'fast track' leadership programme to recruit 'clinicians and external talent to the top jobs'. Health secretary Jeremy Hunt said that this was 'a blueprint for restoring trust in the NHS, reinforcing professional pride in NHS frontline staff and above all giving confidence to patients'. He also stated that there would be a new criminal offence for 'wilful neglect' to hold to account 'those responsible for the worst failures in care'.[10]

The official response to the public inquiry was published

as 'Hard Truths', in two volumes. It declared that targets or finance would *never again be allowed to come before the quality of care*.[11] The CQC was to rate healthcare organisations using *'hard data and soft intelligence'*. Now, only those scoring *'good'* or *'outstanding'* would merit FT status.

It's easy to agree on some things: good care is considerate, correct, careful; bad care is dangerous, erroneous, thoughtless. But just as bad people can do good things, good people can do bad things, especially when circumstances encourage them. A 2013 paper in the *Journal of Medical Ethics* (*JME*) found that in Mid Staffs, *'the means (i.e. quality measurements) became more important than the ends (i.e. good patient care)'*. By using Daniel Kahneman and Amos Tversky's famous thinking fast/slow model to examine what happened, the *JME* found that:

'Since the "the terror of targets" was an ever-present threat, managers avoided adverse risk to themselves by ensuring compliance. This may be understood as a rational, even normal, response. … However, the "frame" to achieve Foundation Trust status may have inclined managers to interpret their function within a consequentialist framework that looked to end-results, but appeared indifferent to the needs of patients.[12] Similarly, for clinicians, they may experience *"cognitive dissonance", where the individual is subject to conflicting ideas. Dissonance is unpleasant. We are naturally motivated to reduce or eliminate it and seek to achieve consonance by "dissonance reduction".*[13]

In other words, professionals with two competing interests – managerial tasks and patient care – may end up failing to speak up for high-quality care when it is easier to agree with enforced managerial targets.

What best leads to effective patient care?

So how can the individuals working in the NHS be helped to do their best work? Does a culture of criminal action for neglect in the NHS make it a better place in which to be a patient?

Not only do we want to ensure that everyone has got good enough care, it's also desirable to be continuously monitoring what is happening because treatments for conditions are always being updated and surgical techniques improved, and we need systems that can constantly utilise the best research in ways that will improve patient care. If something goes wrong in one place in the NHS, it may well be happening in another. It's plain that we would want staff and patients to help flag up problems, see what similar teams elsewhere are doing, compare notes, establish what works well and what needs to change, and how. It's easy to see how this necessitates sharing information and thinking about problems with others.

Do criminal sanctions help? In 2001, a young man was being treated for cancer in Nottingham. As part of his treatment he needed spinal injections of chemotherapy. He was mistakenly injected with vincristine, as a consequence of which he died. The doctor involved was charged with manslaughter and medical negligence, spent 11 months in jail and was eventually sentenced to an eight-month suspended prison sentence.[14] This type of human error had happened almost annually in the preceding 15 years.[15] Would the jail sentence finally stop this mistake from happening? Although it recurred across Europe,[16] it was not until 2014 that the syringe device used was changed to a 'non-Leur' device, physically preventing the same mistake.[17] Nevertheless, the same fatal mistake is possible with other toxic drugs.[18] Why do similar events keep happening? A detailed inquiry placed no blame on the individual doctor but noted that the patient had missed appointments, requested a delay in treatment, and that his treatment had not been ordered, as had been usual, in advance. There were syringes containing different drugs, which looked very similar, with 'no strong visual clues' to tell them apart.[19] One of the doctors had previously worked in a hospital where such dissimilar drugs were stored in different places. An analogy using Swiss cheese helps to explain the cumulation of seemingly small mistakes that led to human disaster: lots of slices of Swiss cheese placed together are unlikely to have one hole that goes all the way from one side to the other. Human error is one hole in one cheese slice. Harms can be stopped from getting all the way through to patients as long as there are enough other layers of safety in the system to compensate.

Criminal sanctions may be effective in inducing fear in humans, and fear can lead to self-preservation. This can mean harmful silence from staff. Francis wrote: '*I have concluded that there is a culture within many parts of the NHS which deters staff from raising serious and sensitive concerns and which not infrequently has negative consequences for those brave enough to raise them*'. Several changes were subsequently made. A statutory Duty of Candour was placed into all CQC registered facilities in England in 2014 and it meant that patients should be told about any harms they had suffered, with a written record being given to them.[20] As promised, the criminal charge was introduced of '*wilful neglect*', with the expectation being that it would be '*easier and more palatable to raise a genuine concern about care standards or patient safety than not*'.[21] '*Genuine errors or accidents*' should not lead to prosecution, whereas acting '*deliberately or recklessly*' could.[22]

Were these measures capable of ensuring mistakes and bad care were less likely to happen? Rather than enabling staff, the legislation may have had the opposite effect. Wilful neglect requires no need to prove harm, and any allegation made about a doctor is prone to lead to their investigation and suspension by the General Medical Council, with one legal advisor stating:

'*The obvious effect it will have is that healthcare workers may not report clinical incidents and near misses for fear of recrimination. That would totally undermine the purpose of the state and, in my view, directly conflicts the new duty of candour legislation. The new legislation risks creating a climate of fear for those on the frontline.*'[23]

Encouraging and protecting informants

An open culture that encourages useful challenge is fundamental to the delivery of high-quality care.[24] The NHS's attitude towards whistleblowers has ranged from mild discouragement to financial pay offs that essentially send out a message to *'keep quiet, go away, and never speak of this again'*.

It's clear from the testimony of whistleblowers that when individuals have spoken up about the consequences for patient care during the management's pursuit of targets they have felt bullied and undermined.[25] The paediatrician Kim Holt, working in the London borough of Haringey, told her hospital managers about the potential for short-staffing and poor record-keeping to compromise patient safety: she was offered a financial settlement to withdraw her complaints. She did not accept, but noted that had action been taken, the killing of Baby P (Peter) by his abusive caregivers would have been far less likely.[26]

This creates a systemic problem of conflicts of interest between the pursuit of targets or financial constraints and clinical care. The hospital lawyers will have given advice designed to protect the hospitals' interests. This is not a system that declarations of transparency or relying on the bravery of whistleblowers to risk their career can systemically overcome. Instead there are competing masters, resulting in staff being disciplined by targets, when those are capable of causing harm. Are there not better ways of reconciling the need to manage systems efficiently with the primary need to put the patients' interests first? I will argue that there are.

Rachel Clarke, *junior doctor*

It's grim.

I come from a family of medics – most are doctors or nurses – and I nearly went in at a conventional age. But I loved English and the Arts, and worked as a documentary-maker. By the time I got to my late 20s, I felt that what I was doing wasn't me. I needed to do medicine. I did my A levels at night, moonlighted at work, and when I was 29 applied to medical school.

Vocation is a word that gets bandied around. I didn't see my decision in those terms at the time, it's only in hindsight I see that's what it was. I was waking up and going into work but not expressing who I was. I was faking it. I always felt a bit fraudulent. Now I have something else. On day one of medical school I felt liberated – it sounds grandiose but it was like the true expression of me, what I was born to be. I didn't need to put on a face, or armour, anymore. I was just learning all this interesting stuff that was worthwhile and would help me do something important, and I had that love all the way through medical school. I loved all of it: the geeky science, the talking to patients, even the really hard things, like seeing someone die or being bereaved. It was all so important; it was what I wanted to be doing.

On day one of being a junior doctor I was beside myself with terror. Like everyone else, you start out and think 'I'm a fraud', 'I can't make any decisions', but at the same time I couldn't believe I was doing this and was finally a doctor. Every day I would cycle in to work, feeling excitement and enthusiasm, doing this thing I just loved.

Right now I'm an ST2 – specialist trainee – working in infectious diseases. I've just applied to palliative care. I've seen things done incredibly well but I've also seen conversations about dying going catastrophically badly. Palliative care has the science of medicine, the hard craft of good diagnosis and making management plans – done well it can make an enormous difference. I'm just drawn to it. To be honest, I'm also pulled away from acute medicine. I've been driven away by the conditions of my work. It's so brutal now.

I'm not seeing things with a rose tint. The first years were frightening, I often felt out of my depth, and I often felt right at the edge or beyond what I was capable of. Long hours, difficult shifts. But my job was a privilege to do. Patients are the absolute reason why you do this job and I felt as though I could do it well. I had this firm, a team – my consultant, registrar and team of juniors. We had solidarity, camaraderie; we looked up to our seniors, and in turn we were respected, guided, mentored. They demonstrated loyalty to us, and wanted to teach and train us. This is an incredibly sustaining part of a young doctor's life in hospital.

Since then it's changed. We are now shift-workers. We have no roots, and no continuity of care for the patients. We have no teams, and we work with different doctors every day. So much has been lost. It's isolating, demoralising, and we are no longer sustained by our relationships with other members of the team. It's always been busy – you don't expect a slack or gentle job. But increasingly the sheer numbers of patients outstrip us by an unsafe degree. It's the worst thing professionally to feel that one of your patients is jeopardised by a lack of standard of care, and you can't do it better because there aren't enough of you. That stress of the working environment is beyond our control. It's soul-destroying. In the last year or so, most hospitals have seen an increase in 'rota gaps'. We are one doctor down just now, so I'm in charge of 50% more patients. I'm working more hours to try and give a safe level of care, waking up worrying at 5 a.m., worrying a patient might slip through the net. It can't carry on indefinitely. This has always been a job requiring stamina and energy, but it is now a job in which the demands can break people. I've seen colleagues who were the very best in the cohort – the ones you thought would be professors and groundbreakers – and have quit; either they can't bear it, or they have taken a levelheaded look at their own future and made the choice to walk away.

We are currently on the edge of a precipice. The government have declared an absolute unwavering intention to impose a contract that 98% of junior doctors have said they will strike against. Our training is in evidence-based medicine – whether a drug or intervention is credible or not. It deeply offends me that we have to listen to the government telling us we've got it wrong – we are trained to do it, and we can sift out soundbites and spin from facts. I don't want to be on a picket line, but I have no choice. The government have misled with statistics, refused to back down, and haven't even defined what a seven-day NHS service is.

Doctors are quite straightforward. They have chosen a job to help people, are driven by simple values – they like to help, and want to do good things with lives. If there is one value more than any other, it's the value of trust. If patients don't trust me, nothing else matters. I am expected to conduct myself in a way that earns trust. Yet the way my government has conducted itself and the spin and misleading way they have used statistics – it's that more than anything else that offends me. They have lost any shred of respect for them I might have had. The language really hurts – calling us 'radicals', using the 'nuclear option' of imposing the contract on us, talking about us as 'militants'. It has made me cry. It's tough enough going into work without having to be spoken about in this manner by your government.

3

The Social Stresses on the NHS

The NHS is based on three principles: *'that it meet the needs of everyone, is free at the point of delivery, and is based on clinical need, not the ability to pay.'* [1]

This declared moral purpose of the NHS is clear and widely agreed. But the NHS does not operate in serene isolation, comfortably insulated from happenings elsewhere in government, society or the world. The NHS has to fill the gaps and take the strain when other parts of public or private services decline or decide not to assist. When social care is underfunded or when public policy is badly formulated and implemented, it is the NHS that often ends up filling the gaps. This safety net of the NHS becomes a trampoline – a lack of social care is met with medical care, and just bounces the persons' problem around, solving nothing, and misdirecting resources.

Medical staff are effectively being asked to sort out poor political policies via the NHS – impossible to do and which merely medicalises a widening range of social problems, from social care, disability and assorted welfare issues to poverty, social inequalities and early years interventions. Furthermore, businesses that profoundly affect public health and have a significant impact on NHS services, such as the alcohol and food industries, contribute to the creation of problems, yet take minimal responsibility, leaving the NHS to sort them out.

Social care

In September 2015, a letter of protest about proposed *'cuts to frontline services'* arrived on the desk of Ian Hudspeth, a county councillor. It read in part:

'*I was disappointed at the long list of suggestions floated in the briefing note to make significant cuts.... from elderly day centres, to libraries, to museums. This is in addition to the unwelcome and counter-productive proposals to close children's centres across the country ... work ... could be done to generate savings in a more creative manner.*'[2]

The reply from the councillor was clear: the council had no other options, having already fired middle managers (losing around 2,800 jobs), changed contracts, frozen pay or given under-inflation pay rises. Services had been merged and physical assets sold off, even though this was '*neither legal, nor sustainable in the long term*'. Although the council was dealing with more older people needing more social support, more children in care and hospitals that were unable to discharge 159 people home because of funding gaps in social care, there was nowhere left to go. While the protestor claimed that the council's spending had '*increased in recent years*', the fact was, replied Hudspeth: '*Our Revenue Support Grant has fallen by almost 50% in the first half of this decade from £122 million in 2011/12 to £62 million in 2015/16, and we expect it to approach zero by 2020. Other funding streams have not kept pace with this, particularly in real terms.*' In addition:

'*... additional functions have been transferred to local authorities since 2009/10. Most notably Public Health as well as new burdens related to the Care Act 2014 and the Health and Social Care Act 2012. ... The Better Care Fund is not new money for the system, there has been £8 million in additional funding for Adult Social Care, but this has been at the expense of funding for NHS Services.*'[3]

The council was having to do more, much more, with less, including delivering public health services. Something had to give. That something was frontline care.

The sender of the letter was David Cameron, the prime minister who had overseen the financial cuts to local councils he was complaining about. Surreally, it seems he simply did not understand that they could not be absorbed without reducing the services available. Local authorities – which commission and pay for social services – have taken hits of 30% of budget in real terms in England and around 24% in Scotland between 2008 and 2015.[4]

Waste in the public sector is morally wrong because it takes resources from others who could benefit: clearly, efficient organisations can offer people more than disorganised ones, which replicate work and spend money on useless tasks. But the budget cuts were upon services that had already made themselves more efficient. A team from Glasgow University, commissioned by the Joseph Rowntree Foundation, wrote: '...*expecting them to deliver the same statutory services and respond to increased demand for some services, represents a massive challenge ... this cannot be achieved solely by "efficiency" changes.*'[5] Deprived areas endured bigger cuts than more affluent ones. Some councils contracted private companies or voluntary organisations to provide welfare advice, even though officers were very aware of the potential for harm: '*We can't do as much as we want to do, and I find that hugely frustrating*', said one. '*We now have another two years ahead and we have taken out the easy savings*', said another.

In November 2015, the Commission on the Future of Health and Social Care in England made a clear statement:

'*We write now out of a deep concern at the many signs that – far from social care and its funding being simplified and improved, as we recommended – the care system itself is instead crumbling around us. That in turn is piling more pressure onto a National Health Service that is struggling both financially and in terms of performance. The government now appears to have no strategy whatever to tackle the rising and pressing needs for social care.*'[6]

Crumbling it may be, but the effect of austerity cuts to social care had been years in the making – and the telling. In the early 2010s, local councils had raised the threshold at which care would be paid for, which meant that people with low or moderate care needs, such as needing help to get dressed or go to the bathroom, were no longer eligible. A daughter described how her mother, who had dementia, was not eligible for social work supported care, so she tried to make sure her mother was safe by means of a fragmented jigsaw of friends, paid help and herself sleeping on the sofa intermittently. But: *'She disappeared regularly, set fire to the kitchen toaster and microwave, had two falls and took an accidental overdose requiring an emergency admission to hospital. It was one of the worst times of my life.'* [7]

It's not difficult to see that inadequate social care has a direct impact on the NHS. Age UK estimated that 800,000 older people have care needs not being met. In 2015 the King's Fund published a report that stated there were more than 5,000 people stuck in hospital because of *'delayed transfers of care'* – unable to go home because they lacked the social support needed to do so. John Appleby, the fund's chief economist, said this was *'clear evidence that cuts to social care budgets are affecting the NHS, as well as reducing services for people that need them'*. [8]

None of the cuts to social care have been subject to trials, of course, and proving cause and effect is impossible. Yet copious evidence exists to show that people in care homes need less hospital and outpatient care. [9] One hospital said that in a week it had 100 patients fit to be discharged but there was nowhere safe for them to go to. [10] Exemplifying this is the tale of 91-year-old Mrs Lee, stuck in hospital for more than 72 days because her care at home would not be taken on by any of the four private companies which her local council commission. Almost 10% of the acute beds in the hospital were needed by people who were medically fit to be discharged but lacked a safe place to go. [11] Even fining local authorities – as has been the case since 1994 – has not made any difference. [12]

Let's be clear what the underlying problem is: providing Mrs Lee's care at home would not turn a profit in the privatised social care sector. Her need for social care is passed over and instead she becomes an NHS responsibility. This is not her fault. It is a double failure of the systems she is trapped in: she is rightly fed up with being away from her husband, and her hospital bed could be better used for someone else. If work is only done when it makes a profit, then the moral values of their work within the interconnected ecosystem they are operating in – namely the NHS – no longer count. The company is not operating as a service, but is operating, as entitled, to make a profit. If hospital wards fill up with people who cannot leave because the social care they need is not available, A&E has nowhere to admit the patients requiring to stay in hospital. The NHS is left to absorb the failures of underfunded and privatised social care. We know that independence is a prized possession of older people,[13] but we don't respect this enough to fund it. What a senseless, short-sighted and cruel way to run our social care and hospital services.

The cuts in social care are especially short-sighted because they have occurred in the context of massive demographic changes in the population. As described in *Living with Dying*,[14] we as a nation are dying older, with more chronic diseases. Frail people need extra support in order to live well and die with dignity. If you are elderly, and struggle to wash, feed or dress yourself because of arthritis, partial-sightedness, stroke, dementia or bronchitis, chances are that you will rely on care support. You may be managing – more or less – independently otherwise, and not be in need of a place in a nursing home. Family members or friends may help, if they are near enough and able to, but if not, the council's social work department will make an assessment of your needs, and then part or fully pay for a carer to visit, up to four times a day. Not getting this right does not get rid of the need for care, it just fails the person and transfers that need onto the NHS. Good social care is not only humane, but there is also evidence that good networks of community care and interventions reduce the need for nursing home care and hospital admissions in the later life of older people.[15] Day centres, homely companionship, activity, meals and safety, were available to 15.3% of people aged over 65 in 2005/6 but only 9.9% in 2012/13.[16]

What effect did that reduction have on the NHS? I know and love our day centres locally. Staff bring patients to us if they suspect a problem, if there has been a fall or a muddle about medication; there is a sense of being part of an extended network of care. Loneliness is a substantive risk factor for earlier death[17] – of a similar order to obesity[18] – and while one can't prove cause and effect (it may be that people are made lonely by poor health, rather than made unhealthier by loneliness), it should surely be considered only kind and decent to ensure that the community can meet the needs of the people inside it, especially marginalised people. We have an NHS safety net, but it is increasingly pressured as the social care safety net is being shredded.

This did not happen unknowingly. In 2011, the King's Fund asked if there was an *an impending crisis*[19] due to social care cuts: *'The consequences are that even fewer people will receive the care and support they need. This will have knock-on effects for people needing NHS care as there will be more emergency admissions to hospital, delayed discharges and longer waits for treatment.'* In 2012, the NHS Confederation said that the cuts to social care were *'unsustainable'* and were costing £200 million annually in delayed discharges.[20]

Mindful of the cuts, in some areas schemes have been trialled to try and treat people in the community rather than admitting them to hospital – *'hospital at home'*, case management, community matrons – but these have not been found to reduce hospital admissions.[21] No matter how well funded social services are, we will still need hospital beds. But hospital beds are being used because there is inadequate social care in the community – to the detriment of people trapped in hospital.

So what happens when there are too few hospital beds? The shift from beds in hospital to the community would logically mean fewer hospital beds were needed. As surgical techniques have improved, fewer days in hospital are needed and bed numbers have plummeted. However, there have been reductions in acute beds and beds classed as *'geriatric'* beds, taking into account both major and community hospitals.[22] The usual *'optimal'* bed occupancy rate is given as 85% (having been 82% in the past[23]) to allow for the time taken to discharge, clean the ward and admit people to hospital –

fuller than this, and there are predictable shortages and crises. This rate has been rising and is now an average of 89.5%.[24] For psychiatric admissions, the bed state is perilous. There are chronic shortages of beds for children who need to be admitted – and when they are, it is often miles from home or into adult beds,[25] which are not designed to care for children. Some areas are spending millions on using private beds, since there is not enough NHS capacity.[26] Delays in finding beds have contributed to tragedies.[27] Doctors described using the law to detain people in order to obtain a bed (which is legally wrong, but perhaps ethically understandable). A random request for bed occupancy over one night in psychiatry found that some hospitals had occupancies of well over 100%,[28] and the overall average was just under 90%.[29]

In the context of robbing hospital Peter to pay community Paul, the bottom line is that both are being stolen from. So what happens? The *'front door'* of the hospital remains open to emergencies, but there are now fewer beds and many of them are needed by people who cannot be discharged home or to a care home because there is not enough social care in the community to do that safely. Consider the Francis Report: the choices made by the austerity agenda enabled, and continue to enable, the same shortcomings in staffing against targets.

Disability and social welfare

Disability and illness are human facts of life. Our welfare system is meant to ensure that people who are already absorbing the effects of disease are not left further disadvantaged. Life as a disabled person is more expensive.

In 2011 I became increasingly worried about the stories I was hearing from people who had been called for medical assessment because of their claim for benefits. Even that term *'claim'* now makes me balk – for people attending for assessments with a doctor, nurse or physiotherapist were to be referred to as *'claimants'*, not *'patients'* according to Atos, the French electronics company that had won the contract to perform disability assessments on behalf of the

Department of Work and Pensions (DWP). Working as a GP, it was increasingly clear to me that Atos was senselessly bureaucratic, hopelessly inaccurate and causing a massive amount of distress for patients and their families. I attended a recruitment evening, noting that the adverts for positions were sold on the idea that doctors could leave on time and be home promptly. Atos were keen to stress there were no targets, but, equally, staff taking too much time would be identified and monitored. I asked the government what evidence the assessments – known as Work Capability Assessments – were based on and what investigation had been done regarding their accuracy and safety. The government couldn't reply. I was referred back to Atos. Atos refused to answer such basic questions, and the Freedom of Information legislation does not apply to private companies, even if they are doing the work of contracts awarded to them by governmental bodies.[30]

The 'tests' that Atos required were superficial and context-less – picking up boxes, for example. The tests were not able to account for common variability in symptoms. For example, people with chronic but fluctuating conditions, such as multiple sclerosis, ME or chronic bronchitis, may be able to do some tasks on one day but not on another. People with mental illness could be assessed by healthcare staff with no particular experience in treating these conditions. In 2013 the Court of Appeal upheld a case brought by the mental health charities Mind and Rethink as well as the National Autistic Society, saying that the tests for Employment and Support Allowance were biased against people with mental health conditions.[31]

Some people struggled to fill out the forms and state their case because of their illness: the reason why people should have received benefits was also the reason why they didn't. The assessments also caused trauma to people being put through a stressful system. The 2013 judgement noted that when one woman 'underwent an assessment in 1995 she was deeply traumatised and despite being awarded IB [Incapacity Benefit], she suffered a relapse and was readmitted to hospital'. In such cases the failings of Atos in the private sector are dealt with in the public sector.

In 2012 the Welfare Reform Bill made its way through parliament. One of the changes enacted was to change Disability Living Allowance (DLA) to Personal Independence Payments (PIP). The stated ideal – that people should have some sort of periodic review rather than a subscription to lifetime allowances – might have seemed reasonable, but the duff outcomes were entirely predictable. People who were clearly going to require long-term support – such as folk with a learning disability, or a congenital problem such as cerebral palsy – were ordered in for review. The government had made a stated claim[32] that reform should result in savings of 20%: this meant the underlying principle was that fewer people would be getting the benefit. The contract was given to private companies Atos and Capita, and was worth £500 million and £140 million, respectively.[33] Enormous delays of six months or more followed. Some of the people waiting for payments will have been terminally ill, and the stress that it caused people who were already living with ongoing medical conditions largely went uncounted. One woman with multiple sclerosis described the process as *guilty until proven innocent*. In the six months between applying for PIP and receiving payments she was made bankrupt and evicted, at one point relying on food banks. Although the payments can be backdated that's of little use if you have no spare money or anyone to lend it to you while you wait.[34] In 2015 the High Court ruled that there had been a *breach of duty on the part of the secretary of state to act without unreasonable delay in determination of the claimant's claims for PIP*.[35] The secretary of state had not upheld his duty to disabled and sick people.

Similarly, the rules around payments of unemployment benefit were so strict as to be cruel. For example, a son was sanctioned – payments withheld – for attending his father's funeral (even though he had told staff at the Job Centre in advance).[36]

The charity Mind described *a lack of understanding of mental health throughout the whole benefits system*, with sanctions being disproportionally applied to mentally ill people, causing additive problems rather than relieving them.[37] This is no wonder, if one considers that many mental illnesses affect people's ability to plan ahead, organise, leave the house or explain oneself to others. External agencies like Citizens' Advice that might be able to help and support people through the process have themselves suffered funding cuts.[38] Back-to-work schemes were not designed or capable of helping mentally ill people to achieve employment: over four-fifths of people Mind surveyed said they felt their mental health was worse as a result of the process.[39] In 2016, the UN Human Rights Committee strongly criticised the UK government for the welfare reforms it had chosen to make, noting that they disproportionately affected the most disadvantaged and marginalised people in our society, making specific reference to the lack of *due process and access to justice* for people who were sanctioned. Ironically, a system meant to help unwell people was actively discriminating against them. We read like a nation festering in meanness.[40]

What has this reform of social welfare done to the NHS? Such enormous changes have been under investigated and largely undocumented. However, one study, published in 2015, sought to relate disability assessments to recordings of antidepressant prescriptions and suicide. This type of study cannot, of course, prove cause and effect, but it did see a firm relationship between them. *'This policy may have had serious adverse consequences'*, the authors wrote,[41] but without such a massive policy being tested for harms in a controlled environment, we will never know for sure.

The *British Medical Journal* (*BMJ*) devoted space in 2015 to questioning the effects of benefit changes on GP workload. Three-quarters of GPs had noted some form of increase in appointments related to benefits problems, especially (and predictably) those working in inner cities. The change to Housing Benefit (dubbed the *'bedroom tax'*) – where benefits were reduced when people had unoccupied rooms – was an especial problem for people who used a spare room for overnight stays for carers or relatives helping to look after someone, and resulted in debt for many who did not have the option of moving to a smaller house or flat. People sought help from GPs, not only for stress but also documentation to assist in claims. As one GP put it, *'It's a patient contact that's generated that would otherwise not have happened. It's a ten-minute consultation, 15 minutes writing a report and planning it, and the secretary's time'*. When multiplied by thousands of instances across the UK a sizeable dent is soon made in the amount of available GP appointments. Surveys carried out by the *BMJ* make it clear that at least part of the pressure on GP appointments was likely due to the burden of the reformed welfare system.[42] The reforms were fundamentally unfair on the people subjected to them and the health service coping in the aftermath.

Poverty and social inequalities

There are some people who think that poverty does not exist in modern Britain. They are wrong. We may have moved on from slums and childhood labour; instead, we have families trying to live on unstable, zero-hours contracts, paying high prices for fuel, in damp, overcrowded housing and without nearby safe space for children to play. Chronic disease and disability places vulnerable families at a high risk of social exclusion. Although trying to define poverty in relative terms is very difficult,[43] Oxfam say that one in five of our population lives in poverty.[44]

Food bank use has sharply increased. One provider, the Trussell Trust, described how just under 350,000 people used one of their food banks in 2012/13 which increased to over 900,000 in 2013/14.[45] The number one reason for people attending was benefit delays; the second, low income. The workers at the Trussel Trust cited benefit sanctions as a major issue, and the stories are horrendous: a family of four, whose father has a mental illness and a mother who cares for her own mother, who has Parkinson's. The family was sanctioned because the father was given the wrong address to go for an Employment and Support Allowance (ESA, the replacement for IB) appointment. They ended up living on £50 a week for 12 weeks: *'I had gone without to feed my kids, and would go without again ... I never thought I'd be in this situation.'* Another person who was sanctioned when he missed an appointment was in hospital being treated for a heart attack.[46]

I've spoken to many who have felt humiliated by the process of benefit claims – shame at being assumed to be guilty of *'cheating'* the system. For people who have a life-impairing or life-shortening illness this simply isn't fair. The NHS takes the impact as the – privatised – benefits system fails. Firstly, through the impact of the paperwork required to furnish the process. Secondly, being used as a referral or redirection agency for people who are in crisis and without enough food. Thirdly, dealing with the physical and mental stress which many people put through this system suffer. And then to deal with the long-term consequences of children growing up in poverty.

Public health researchers wrote in the *BMJ* in 2015 that while further welfare reform would mean pensioners and those without children would be better off, lone parents and families with children would be worse off.[47] Another group of researchers calculated that this would result in 200,000 more children being brought up in poverty, a figure that could rise further over the length of the policy.[48] Writing in the *BMJ*, they noted how children aged five and living in the greatest poverty are a year, developmentally, behind their peers; and children growing up in homes of financial hardship are at higher risk of depression and anxiety.[49] There is also a clear gradient where deaths in babies are more common in poorer families.[50] So 5.2 out of every 1,000 children born to families working in the professional classes will die as infants compared to nine born into families working in the lowest paying jobs. Infant mortality is falling overall, but such a clear distinction of life-chances at birth signals social inequality at work. The most common operation in children aged between five and nine is the removal of decayed teeth,[51] and the poorest children have more tooth decay.[52] Children and adults from deprived backgrounds use A&E services more.[53]

As we age, we accumulate more long-term disease, but if we are poor our chronic disease diagnoses – like chronic bronchitis or heart disease – happen on average 10–15 years earlier than they do for the better-off.[54] Mental and physical ill-health frequently ride together.[55] Poverty slowly and inexorably steals life and healthy years – and, of course, lifespan overall. Men and women in the poorest areas live an average of 19.3 years and 20.1 years less than those in the richest, respectively.[56] This well-known and repeatedly confirmed fact should be considered a scandal in plain sight. Yet it is a fact so absorbed and accepted that it is dismissed as inevitable and unfixable; there is no fierce challenge to *'the way things are'.* Instead, policies are launched with little regard for who might be harmed. Charities and voluntary organisations are left to attempt to plaster into the cracks and gaps which open and widen. And all this has a direct effect on the role of the NHS. It cannot fix health inequalities caused by a lack of money, which is the gateway into security of food, clothing, childcare, self-care and accommodation. Instead, the NHS acts as an army doctor does in war, patching people up only to throw them back out again to be injured.

Poor people die younger.[57] Julian Tudor Hart reported it in 1971,[58] when he wrote: *'Medical services are not the main determinant of mortality or morbidity; these depend most upon standards of nutrition, housing, working environment, and education, and the presence or absence of war.'* In 1980, the Black Report made the same thing clear.[59] And Michael Marmot has repeatedly pointed it out through his career; as he put it in 2010: *'Health inequalities result from social inequalities. Action on health inequalities requires action across all the social determinants of health.'*

What are these social inequalities? There are numerous models that attempt to explain why this pervasive effect of poverty equalling earlier death occurs (for example, less money equals a bigger risk of damp homes, leading to an increased risk of respiratory disease, or an increased chance of being born to a mother who smokes, leading to poor growth in the womb). There are likely to be many interdependent explanations, from ongoing financial and social stress, such as the uncertainty of benefits claims), poor housing and unemployment, to what has been termed *'food deserts'* (an inability to get fresh food locally) or the relationship between income and smoking.

The critical question is what has to happen to make things better. There is a 20-year gap in life expectancies between the richest and poorest. Marmot has written, with justified fury:

'There would be about 202,000 fewer premature deaths each year if everyone in Britain had the low level of mortality of those with university education (which was less than 10% of the population when the people dying today were of student age). That is about 500 deaths a day. It is a calamity for each of us, potentially, and a tragedy for the nation. If this toll resulted from a pollutant, people would take to the streets demanding action. We should demand action. The cause is inequality in the conditions in which people are born, grow, live, work and age; and inequities in power, money and resources that give rise to this inequality.' [60]

Marmot goes on to point out that in more than 80% of low-income households, at least one adult was working. Social inequalities aren't caused by laziness, or people choosing to have a poorer quality of health. Instead, they arise from circumstances partially or completely out of people's control, which have small, cumulative effects on their life chances, possibilities, directions and, ultimately, quality of life and time of death. Caring for relatives, going to an overstretched school, having a lack of good childcare, living in an area of greater pollution – all these add together and translate into inequalities becoming deadly. All of these factors are outside the health service's control. The NHS will deal with the consequences of health inequalities. It cannot cure them. In Scotland, we are encouraged to treat people living in areas of greater social deprivation earlier with cholesterol-lowering pharmaceuticals. This is literally attempting to treat poverty with drugs. Although the intention may be honourable, it does not fix the cause of the problem – even if people did faithfully take the tablets for the prescribed decades, it would not be enough to overturn all the consequences of inequality. It is a medicalisation of poverty.

Michael Marmot and his team argue that, in the US, *'living wages'* – a minimum income paid per hour – are *'associated with significant improvements in life expectancy, self-rated health, depression, alcohol consumption, activity-limiting illnesses and a fall in mortality'.*[61] Many *'mindfulness'* programmes have been rolled out in schools in the UK to supposedly *'help build resilience'* and *'reduce stress'.* I wonder why we are comfortable spending money on this and not, say, on free school meals, or ensuring that parents are not having to cope with the stress and uncertain income of zero-hours contracts or benefits sanctions in the first place. There is evidence that small amounts of money can enable homeless people to find permanent accommodation.[62] In the US, a regular non-means tested income to disadvantaged Native Americans was associated with benefits to children that were still detectable a quarter of a century later.[63] In Canada, a minimum income was associated with a reduction in hospital use, admissions for mental illness, and accidents and injuries.[64]

One might reasonably expect that medical organisations in the UK – Royal Colleges, medical charities or NHS federations – would therefore pay at least the living wage. Many do not,[65] with some using the excuse that subcontractors – particularly for cleaning – were not direct employees. If such well-funded, financially secure organisations – and those most likely to know the evidence about income and health – are not ensuring that the most poorly paid are at least remunerated to minimum standards, then god help us all. When the cheapness of a contract is prioritised before the reasonable treatment of staff, the latter bear the personal cost of the bargain contract. It is a disgrace that hospital cleaners are being paid less than the London Living Wage and have had to resort to striking to draw attention to it.[66] Cleaners are integral to a well-run health system. Whose moral values are we riding on?

Early years intervention

Sure Start Children's Centres were a strategy to tackle social disadvantage, announced in 1998. These were meant to level out inequalities by providing support, financial assistance, childcare and learning to preschool children. A cross-departmental governmental strategy had tried to work out what best to do, and in the words of the then Treasury Deputy Director Norman Glass:

'... a number of academics and campaigning groups with an interest in children's services had made their views known. It was evident that there was a considerable expertise in the policy community which was eager to play a part in the development of the policy and that the sensible way forward was to make as much use as possible of this expertise.'

Even better: ministers agreed that they would hold seminars with the academic community and 'commission a review of what the evidence said about what worked'. It was a 'prime example of joined up government and evidence-based policymaking'.[67] Evidence making a policy – exciting stuff! However, there was no widespread randomised controlled trial (which would have been perfectly possible), a fact which the government was accused of vetoing[68] and which would have made later evaluations more reliable.[69] However, some smaller randomised trials were done in Wales as the scheme was rolled out, which found that it did reduce behavioural problems in children.[70] Money was poured in. Later analysis of Sure Start centres found there were benefits for children, including better relationships with caregivers, and more learning opportunities for children.[71] Over a million families might have been using the Sure Start centres, but the coalition government of 2010 removed the centres' ring-fenced budget,[72] which led to plans for centres to close down (entirely, in Newcastle, or almost entirely – 54 down to ten centres in Staffordshire).

In 2016 a report was quietly published[73] that found that

children using the centres had more stable home lives and better social skills, and this led to better mental health for parents. Families appreciated these centres and more vulnerable families had good access to them. However, austerity cuts reduced their funding, and, as a consequence, could only offer less care.[74] The Sure Start policy was popular intervention with evidence of long-term impact, which rationally could have improved the health of people who were most likely to die young. And yet the funding is, at the time of writing, insecure and floundering.

Public Health and the NHS

Public Health is healthcare for the masses: here the population is the patient and policy is the medicine. Strong public health should enable mass interventions to be funded and run in ways that cut inequalities and improve quality of life – from clean water and sanitation to vaccination programmes. Public health should be a practice of evidence-based medicine, even while operating in a complex intertwining of politics, industrial influences and financial constraints.

Take the plain packaging of cigarettes. In 2008 there was experimental evidence showing that packaging played a key role in the perception of the effects of cigarette products.[75] By 2011, the coalition government said it would consult on the evidence for plain packs. But it did not – as hoped and expected – make plans for a law to proceed in 2013.[76] Instead, the government proceeded to various consultations. However, there were many reports of lobbying, including from the 'election guru' to the Conservative Party, Lynton Crosby. His consultancy had tobacco companies as clients and he was found to have lobbied on behalf of them just a few weeks before taking up his new election position in 2012.[77] As the date for a vote in parliament on standardised cigarette packaging drew near, tobacco companies paid for wraparound advertising in Westminster magazines, having previously paid for MPs to attend events from the opera *La traviata* to the Chelsea Flower Show as well as pop concerts.[78]

As the UK flim-flammed, Australia passed new plain pack law in 2012. By 2013, in Australia, it was found that customers were less likely to find plain-packaged cigarettes appealing, and more inclined to want to give up smoking.[79] Nor were unintended consequences detected, such as the market being flooded by cheaper cigarettes.[80] It was clear by 2015 that the drop in cigarette use was ongoing, with children being more likely to delay starting smoking.[81] The UK government, still consulting in 2014, found in an independent review:

'There is very strong evidence that exposure to tobacco advertising and promotion increases the likelihood of children taking up smoking ... [it is] ... highly likely that standardised packaging would serve to reduce the rate of children taking up smoking and implausible that it would increase the consumption of tobacco.' [82]

This could therefore be reasonably seen as a useful public health intervention: after all 17% of all adult deaths are attributable to smoking.[83] It was noted that most of the opposing submissions cited science that was either irrelevant to the issue of plain packaging or was of poor quality.[84] In May 2015, legislation was finally passed to commence plain packaging from May 2016. However, the tobacco industry responded by launching a legal claim at the High Court to protest that it infringed *'property rights'*.[85]

The alcohol industry

From William Hogarth's etching *Gin Lane* (1751) onwards, there is a long social history of alcohol not just providing pleasure, conviviality and fun, but also harm. The damage has direct impact on the NHS, including treatment for poisoning and addiction, and the consequences of domestic and street violence.

The NHS is not just there for bad luck – the cancer that arrives in the chastely living, non-smoker person who exercises three times a week and who eats plenty of greens. No – the NHS will treat skiing injuries and footballers' injured knees; it will prescribe drugs with the sole purpose of enabling people to have sex; and you can get paracetamol, which is available cheap and over the counter, on prescription. So why shouldn't drinkers – who pay a large amount into the NHS through tax on their alcohol – be entitled to a share of NHS services if they find that alcohol turns them into a patient?

I agree that the NHS should be just as available to people with a drink-related need as to any other. It is as foolish to judge who *'deserves'* NHS care as it is to decide who the *'unlucky'* person with cancer is (for are we sometimes going to decree that some cancers are justly deserved?). It would be nonsense to restrict NHS care by judging whether an illness is *'self-inflicted'* or adequately *'deserving'*. A libertarian trust underlies the principle of *'free at the point of need'*. Indeed, the risks of illness are often determined by factors outwith our control. For example, there is a strong genetic influence on alcohol addiction.[86] Similarly, people living in deprived neighbourhoods are at an increased risk of binge drinking.[87]

As stated previously, from 2010 more people have been going to, and waiting longer in, A&E. In 2003/4, 16.5 million people went to A&E, compared to 22.3 million ten years later.[88] One study from Newcastle found that alcohol played a role in between 12% and 15% of those cases presenting for attention in A&E.[89] The rate of increase is enormous: between 2005/6 and 2013/14, the amount of people admitted as an emergency with an alcohol-related condition more than doubled.[90]

I have no wish to stop people enjoying alcohol. I do, though, have a wish to ensure the sustainability of the NHS. And there are evidence-based policies that could help to limit the damage caused by alcohol. There is nothing new in legislating to regulate potentially harmful substances: like the 1751 Gin Act.[91] In my local supermarket there are many alcoholic drinks available at less than the price of a carton of orange juice or cola. In 2009 the *'Sheffield Studies'* had made it clear that minimum pricing for alcohol was likely to have a beneficial effect in the UK, and in 2010 the House of Commons Health Select Committee recommended minimum alcohol pricing but no action was forthcoming.

Elsewhere in 2010, in Saskatchewan, Canada, the law was used to set the price of alcohol – to around 50p per unit strength. Taking before-and-after data, the effect of the 10% rise in costs was a 16% reduction in drinking.[92] Drink driving fell by 19%[93] and crime overall by 9%. There were decreases in alcohol-related hospital attendances by around 9%. Considering that there were over 140,000 alcohol-related admissions during this time, this is a substantial drop[94] – and if the alcohol consumption is reduced, as expected, in the longer term, fewer alcohol-related conditions will develop, from liver disease to breast, throat or bowel cancer. Furthermore, after the minimum price was introduced, deaths purely due to alcohol dropped quickly, a reduction still found at the end of the study.[95]

Any such policy change is also capable of doing harm – for example, could people with alcoholism change to cheaper but more harmful substances (such as methanol)? However, this hasn't been demonstrated.[96] Would a minimum price affect more lower-paid people than higher-paid ones? Yes, but the difference is likely to be small: 0.5% in lower-paid groups versus 0.3% increase in grocery bills for higher-paid groups.[97] Here is a policy with a decent amount of proof, which has shown a strong association of a beneficial effect on both citizens and the health service.

Extensive modelling work in the UK predicts much the same useful effect from a minimum alcohol price.[98] So why hasn't it been done? In 2015, Wales set out plans to introduce minimum pricing,[99] and in 2012 Scotland passed the necessary legislation with cross-party support, but that was then challenged in law by the Scotch Whisky Association.[100] This challenge is going through the European courts and has not been resolved as this book goes to print. Models suggest that for every year that implementation is delayed, at least 1,600 hospital admissions could have been avoided.[101] It may be no surprise that the alcohol industry is unhappy with this policy, but it is the NHS meantime that is taking the strain.

In 2010, the House of Commons Health Select Committee had stated: '*It is time the Government listened more to the Chief Medical Officer and the President of the Royal College of Physicians and less to the drinks and retail industry. If everyone drank responsibly the alcohol industry would lose 40% of its sales and some estimates are higher. In formulating its alcohol strategy, the Government must be more sceptical about the industry's claims that it is in favour of responsible drinking.*'[102]

Health secretary Andrew Lansley set out a '*responsibility deal*' with the alcohol industry, which rested on '*nudges*' rather than legally enforceable terms.[103] It was claimed that industry would effectively regulate itself, a billion units of alcohol could be taken out of circulation through co-operation, and the health of the nation would therefore improve. Yet data from the Health and Social Care Information Centre has found rises in alcohol-related hospital admissions: in 2014/15 there were an estimated 1,059,210 hospital admissions due to alcohol, 5% more than in 2012/13.[104]

In 2012, however, the government declared that it would set a minimum price for alcohol, calculating that it would save 900 alcohol-related deaths every year.[105] Then it all went wonky. Think tanks, some sponsored by industry, produced reports decrying minimum pricing. Lobbying – much of it financed by the alcohol industry – took place on a frequent basis and often went un-minuted. A political campaign adviser to the prime minister was reported to urge him to ditch controversial policies in advance of the forthcoming election. On the day before the summer 2013 parliamentary recess – thus minimising the time for effective scrutiny – minimum pricing for alcohol was withdrawn because there was, allegedly, not enough '*concrete evidence*' for it.[106] It's difficult not to conclude that the alcohol industry had played this policy game, set and match. In Scotland, an act of Parliament was passed in 2012 which would set a minimum price on alcohol. It had cross party support, but a challenge by the Scotch Whisky Association has meant it is still not enacted in 2016.[107]

And, of course, the NHS continues to take the hit from those patients attending with alcohol-related ailments.

The food industry

I am sceptical of the clean eating movement, and I don't own a juicer. Nevertheless: the food industry has created avoidable pressure for the NHS and it has been inadequately challenged.

In 2016, NICE proposed to contract GPs to measure the body mass index (BMI) of all their patients, saying: *'Calculating BMI will enable primary care to identify people who are overweight and obese, which can then lead to primary care playing a key role in weight management through assessing risk and morbidity, and facilitating access to weight management support.'*[108] According to Chief Medical Officer Dame Sally Davies: *'It absolutely is a GP's duty to let patients know if they or their children are overweight, because it is the precursor of such dreadful ill health. We can't afford to ignore it.'*[109] But there is no secret intervention GPs know that can make people lose weight in the long term. In fact, for every 1,000 people invited to Weight Watchers (a long-term lower-calorie eating plan), only ten will have maintained their goal weight five years later.[110] There is no good research evidence about what weight-loss programme is suitable for pregnant woman[111] and proven interventions that help prevent childhood obesity involve healthy school meals and time for exercise, not doctor's appointments.[112]

My point is that doctors cannot be responsible for the prevention of obesity, which is not a problem that can be solved inside consulting rooms. Obesity comes with a long history of ineffective and dangerous medication; in the 1930s, amphetamines ('*speed*') were prescribed, causing addiction.[113] In 2010, sibutramine was banned after it was found to cause heart attacks, while also not being very effective.[114] Indeed, only bariatric surgery is notably effective in the long term,[115] but it comes with significant side effects, and in the UK it is only available to a limited number of people.

The coalition government's response to rising obesity was another *'responsibility deal'* set up in 2011. Again, the *'working together'* rhetoric was supposedly going to ensure improvements, all done voluntarily.[116] *'Big food'* would cut calories and therefore stop obesity; this would enhance their trustworthiness and reputation, and government wouldn't have to create new laws. Win–win. By 2015, researchers examined the effect of the industry's pledges on calorie reduction and were not able to find evidence of new strategies. The most effective known strategies to cut calorie intake (such as a reduction in advertising or pricing policies) weren't taken up. Rather than reducing calories, as Andrew Lansley had said the deal would (*'it is a great step in the right direction and will help millions of us eat and drink fewer calories'*[117]), the researchers found that calorie intake had actually continued to increase.[118] Analysis of how much sugar is taken home in shopping baskets shows increases over the life of the policy,[119] while the government's own statistics show a slow decrease in calorie intake overall (including that from sugar) – but this is taken from surveying selected households rather than actual shopping data.[120]

I think it is fair to say that the effect of the voluntary deal is invisible. An illusion of *'doing something'* is created such that policymakers believe the problem is virtually solved. People working for large food companies described their signing up to the responsibility deal as also about reputation, and disclosed that often the changes would have happened without signing up. Benefits of doing so included *'access to government'*.[121] I saw a lot of rehabilitation. For example, the soft drinks company Coca-Cola set up partnerships with local councils worth £20 million to offer exercise schemes in local parks – a fact that was advertised widely with the company's logo included, with permanent posters in the parks themselves. *'Our research reveals that there is a £2.1 billion opportunity to grow the soft drinks category, including £793 million of incremental sales that can be unlocked by delivering just one more soft drink "moment" per household per week'* declared the company, which meant £20 million was small change for ingraining itself into local life.[122]

In the US, Coke had stood accused of using paid experts to *'product place'* their drinks into health columns. The Global Energy Balance Network, which promoted the idea that exercise was more important than diet in preventing obesity, was funded by Coca-Cola – a fact that was not declared on its website.[123] Academics who have accepted consultancy funding from Coca-Cola have challenged studies which have suggested that Coca-Cola is related to poorer health,[124] despite that rarest of things – a medical journal deciding that *'there is sufficient scientific evidence that decreasing sugar-sweetened beverage consumption will reduce the prevalence of obesity and obesity related diseases'.*[125] (More usually, research concludes *'more research must be done'.*) The Coca-Cola product glacéau vitaminwater was widely advertised as *'nutritious'* before the Advertising Standards Authority decided that the 23 g of sugar contained in one drink was a quarter of the daily recommended amount.[126] These are not healthy products: they are linked to obesity.[127]

In Mexico, in 2013, a tax (roughly 10%) was placed on sugary drinks with the intention of reducing consumption and hence obesity. After the tax there was a clear 12% reduction in purchases of sugary drinks.[128] So should a similar *'soda tax'* be rolled out in the UK? Other evidence suggests that it would work.[129] There is a strong case for trials to be done. Yet it is also clear that there is an entanglement of industry professionals, grants, academic papers, consultancy fees, promotional activities and government lobbying.[130] It is impossible to know whether these represent conflicts of interest that have changed the nature of public health in the UK. But is such a tangled web the best way to make evidence-based policy that is capable of cutting through bias and doing the best thing for public health? In the budget of 2016, George Osborne pledged a *'sugar tax'* on soft drinks,[131] which prompted a fall in share prices and immediate hostility from the drinks industry.[132]

Are the choices that government makes led by industry and the professionals supporting them? For if the policy fails, it is – again – the NHS that has to pick up the pieces. There are ongoing academic arguments about whether the taxation raised from trading in tobacco or alcohol offsets the costs they cause the NHS. Yet in many ways this is moot. This taxation is not simply to meet the costs caused by these products: it is treated as core funding in the bigger sum along with taxation from many other sources, and is not ring fenced. Were sales of these products to fall, taxation would simply be raised from other means. Nor is this simply an equation of financial cost: it creates avoidable pressures in the NHS and human harm.

There is worrying evidence that commercial interests are embedded in public health politics. Plans for policies with cross-party agreement and with reasonable evidence go contested over years in the courts. But there is a deep illogic in public health policymaking. In 2015, NICE recommended that GPs should ask all their older patients about home heating. There is no doubt that cold homes are bad for health. But it was the government that, in 2012, axed the universally popular Warm Homes, Healthy People project, which helped with emergency boiler repairs and heating. It was a popular project because it was flexible and placed people's needs before bureaucratic ones.[133] Better-heated homes result in fewer doctor's appointments and fewer symptoms of asthma in children,[134] and a Cochrane review (a high-quality appraisal of all the evidence on the topic) found that improvements to housing led to health benefits.[135] The inconsistencies in use of evidence to make decisions are stark and incompatible with a sustainable NHS.

Interview

Eric Rose, retired GP principal

*I qualified in 1968, and always intended to go into general practice.
I started in Norfolk in 1972, then went to Aylesbury where I was for
21 years. I had a break as the Local Medical Committee secretary
for five years. I missed the patients but got lots of ideas about how
practices could be run, and got the chance to set up a new practice
in Milton Keynes – we started in 1998 with no patients and I retired
in 2008 with 12,500 patients and six partners.*

*My first 21 years were really pushing GP [general practice]
forward. We arranged a lot of meetings with other GPs locally,
where we'd pick one another's brains and try out new ideas. We
would all agree to do an audit in our practice – what we were
prescribing for something, for example – come back, discuss what
we found, compare our results, think about why they were different.
I thought it was good as we wanted to do it and we thought it was
the right thing to do – we weren't paid money to do these things.*

*The 1966 contract allowed us to expand and grow, and although
there were financial incentives, they were monies for services, like
vaccinations or cervical screening – not targets. After 1990 (when
Kenneth Clarke imposed a new contract) things started to get more
difficult, with increasing political interference in the day-to-day
work of general practice. This happened under governments of both
main parties. Then what went most wrong with general practice
was to do with the 2004 contract. Even though I was in the General
Practitioners Committee [GPC], who were in charge of negotiating
the contract with the Department of Health, I argued against many
aspects of the contract because it tied a lot of funding to QOF
(Quality and Outcomes Framework) activity and tied income to
the Carr-Hill formula, which was totally flawed.* *

The 2004 contract also got rid of the commitment for GPs

---

* *The Carr-Hill formula is used to weight money paid to GPs
per patient, varying with factors such as age, rurality and
patients in nursing homes.*

to cover their patients 24 hours a day, 365 days a year. I was one of the lead campaigners over the 'out of hours' [OOH] issue. In 1992 I proposed the motion to commit the GPC to work towards getting rid of the 24-hour commitment. In 1996, there was a partial change in the rules and a small amount of extra funding. As a result of this, GPs almost everywhere were setting up or had set up GP OOH co-operatives. By and large they were very good. They were run by GPs who knew what they were doing, ensured patients got seen and wanted them dealt with properly – because, frankly, we didn't want to hand over to a night-time service who didn't provide a quality service, because the next day you'd have to pick up the mess. GPs being personally responsible for providing round-the-clock cover became increasingly unsustainable, partly because of increasing workload and also because there were more and more part-time principals (partners) in GP. Some doctors didn't want to become GPs because of the heavy night-time commitment. When I started work, it was in an area where we did our own on call. I chose this deliberately as I wanted to give complete care to my patients. Sometimes, if I had been up in the night, there was an hour between surgeries to take a nap. Going out to help someone in the middle of the night could be a pleasure, although I still got tired the next day. Over the next few years, it changed. Daytime surgeries got busier, family life had to be planned around the on call rota. My wife had to be home by 6 p.m. to answer the phone and during weekends couldn't leave the house at all. I was on call and unable to visit my wife in hospital after our second child was born when my son had a serious accident at home. I was trying to staunch his bleeding with one hand while holding the phone in the other, trying to find someone else to do my duty. It was unsustainable.

There was another main reason why the changes to out of hours got pushed through. The government had the notion that they could do it better, and that they would somehow organise so-called 'unscheduled' care by co-ordinating ambulance service, A&E, GP OOH service and nurses in walk-in centres and direct patients appropriately. In the end, the Primary Care Trusts

[PCT] – who were then put in charge of commissioning night and weekend cover – got the same amount of money, about £9,000 per GP to arrange care. But some PCTs used it for other purposes, not just out of hours care, and put cheaper people in the front line. Of course, nurses can do some of the things that GPs do – but the idea that you could simply slot a nurse into work done by GPs and hope it would be as efficient is just wrong. I studied this locally and found that nurses in the walk-in centre were nearly three times as expensive per consultation as GPs and took longer.

The paperwork simply increased. We had ridiculous things, like, say, asking a community nurse if she could do something – we had to do a four-page form. Instead of my being able to ring a consultant and say I am a bit worried about this patient, can you slot them in at a clinic? – and they would know me – I had to fill in a form instead. We relied on QOF points, as we were a practice with a lot of young people and a low Carr-Hill funding result, so we spent a lot of time chasing people to get the last few QOF points. That kind of box-ticking inhibited proper general practice. The targets that we were set seemed to make care worse, not better.

Despite all that, I still got great satisfaction from my job – working with patients, helping through my knowledge, being able to advise, and sometimes from experience pick up things that hadn't been noticed already – but I was also dissatisfied by trying to cope with a rising sense of workload and an increased demand and sense of entitlement on the part of some patients. Most of my patients were brilliant, but this was a new city – Milton Keynes – and many new patients had no family network. Anxiety was stoked by the press: for example, make sure that every childhood fever is not meningitis. I spent a lot of time reassuring people that their child did not have meningitis – in fact, I never saw a case of meningococcal sepsis in my career. I miss my patients. But I don't miss the 11-hour days.

4

The Evidence-Based NHS

How do we know what works? The ancient Greeks developed a theory that the human body consisted of four basic 'humours', which were blood, phlegm, black bile and yellow bile. For Hippocrates (460–370 BC), human health depended on a balance between the humours and illness was simply a disruption of this balance. Galen of Pergamum (AD 129–200) declared that blood was the most important humour, and cupping, leeching and bloodletting became common therapeutic medical practices.[1] This theory survived until just a few centuries ago. In 1685, when King Charles II had a stroke, he was drained of almost 700 ml of his blood. His physicians apparently fled the scene when he died.[2]

If a patient didn't improve, it was considered to be due to a lack of the treatment, and if death resulted, doctors argued for more bloodletting done sooner. And so bloodletting continued during the American Civil War and during cholera outbreaks in the 19th century. It was given to popes and princes as well as the common man and woman.

It's obvious to us now that bloodletting as a treatment for stroke or infection is not just useless but dangerous. It took until the mid-1800s for arguments to surface asking the crucial question – does it work? Dr John Hughes Bennett (1812–1875), a doctor from Edinburgh who had worked across Europe, performed laboratory research to test the practice. He concluded that removing blood from a fevered person was likely to be dangerous. Younger than most of the medical establishment, he lectured medical students that scientific knowledge *'was silently revolutionising the study of medicine'.*[3] Of the fallout, medical historian John Harley Warner noted: *'Most Edinburgh medical men maintained that the proper role of science was to explain and legitimise – but not test or guide – medical practice; they further held that science should be consistently subordinated to bedside observation even in formulating theories to explain therapeutic actions.'* [4]

In other words: expert opinion was key to what doctors did. If your elders – and therefore betters – supported bloodletting, you, junior to them, must follow suit. Doctors were not to test their treatments. They were simply expected to administer and possibly to explain them – to fit their theory to what observably happened. An observer, biased towards his own treatment, is far less likely to think: has my treatment killed or harmed my patient? This *'observer bias'* is yet to be resolved. Iain Chalmers, now the editor of the James Lind Library, described his own realisation as follows: *'I had been harming my patients by relying on "eminence-based" rather than "evidence-based" guidance.'* [5]

James Lind joined the Royal Navy as a surgeon's mate in 1738, after his medical training. His book *A Treatise of the Scurvy* was published in 1753. In the book he examines theories as to the causes of scurvy and describes his experiments on the sailors using different treatments.[6] For his time, his approach was distinctly refreshing. He reviewed the evidence, constructed a theory and tested it. The online library named after him documents the evolution of *'fair tests'.*[7]

Of course, evidence by itself has no moral quality. It would be possible to study the most effective ways to maim, kill or harm in healthcare. When we generate evidence, we also need to have a moral purpose, such as aiming to add to the quality and quantity of life. It's not good enough to say that something is *'evidence-based'* and use this phrase as a justification for using it; does this evidence help us to provide something useful and of meaning for the people who are intended to use it? Core to the *'morality'* of research has been a historical failure to look for things of use to patients. So for example, people with rheumatoid arthritis were not so keen to find out what treatments improved various blood counts or even pain, despite a large amount of research doing just this. Instead they wanted treatments to improve their chances of feeling less tired. Most modern research was not investigating the best treatments for what they wanted to know.[8] If we don't do fair tests of whether we are doing the right thing, we do harm: and if we do tests which aren't capable of answering the questions that needed answered, we do harm.

It is, therefore, common sense that non-evidence-based medicine can kill and maim. Exactly the same is true of non-evidence-based NHS policy, which harms people and wastes resources. The NHS should be making policy based on the aims of its moral constitution (care according to need, free at the point of use). That means doing policymaking with the full knowledge that poor decisions create harms. It means investigating uncertainties properly, with thorough systematic reviews of what is currently known, and proper trialling and testing. And for this we need a culture in which we actively look for and consider harms; an understanding of what evidence can and cannot do; and an appreciation of 'opportunity costs' and unintended consequences.

Fair tests – randomised controlled trials (RCT)

So, how do we know how much of the £116 billion spent annually on the NHS is a modern equivalent to bloodletting?[9] What do we do that works, and what does not work? We could double, triple or quadruple our spending on health yet waste it all if we spend it on things that don't work. So what wastes time, money and life? What helps patients to live better? What increases bureaucracy without improving quality? Does it help patients to choose the best care option if individual surgeon's death rates are published? Can a patient be safely seen by a nurse or physiotherapist instead of a doctor? Does an expensive new hip replacement provide years of pain-free walking, or does it simply cost more with no added value? We will only know the answers to any of these questions if we use 'fair tests' of new treatments or ways to organise ourselves. This is simple: don't waste time, money and staff. Don't do things that don't work. We do not systematically do this, and the result is waste: in money, time and lives. A lack of appreciation in the NHS for the need for decent science has done untold harms, as I will demonstrate. But many of these harms are hardly obvious without fair tests.[10]

Why do we need fair tests? Take one clinical problem: antibiotics. A person receiving antibiotics for a cold will note that the cold gets better after taking the antibiotics. Were we to look at that evidence alone, it would seem that antibiotics worked because common colds would get better after a week of taking them. Look, they work! Doctors would feel justified in prescribing them. Patients would see that their symptoms were relieved after popping the penicillin, but there would be no red flags signalling what we know because of science: colds get better anyway, whether or not antibiotics are taken.

The scientific method gave us this knowledge. Ideally, one would clone oneself to give two batches of identical subjects. One group would take the antibiotic and the other would not. Then the two outcomes could be compared. In the absence of human clones, a randomised controlled trial (RCT) is done instead. RCTs are the lynchpins of knowing whether medicine kills or cures – or, more commonly, where the balance of risk and benefit lies. Two groups of people, as evenly matched as possible, are compared. The only difference between the groups is the treatment under test. When these 'controlled' trials have been done – 'control' describing the comparative group who aren't given the treatment under test – we can see quite clearly that antibiotics don't make a difference to the duration of a cold.[11] Worse, antibiotics cause side effects like diarrhoea, and bacteria ultimately become resistant to antibiotics placed in common use. Antibiotics are not just useless treatments for colds and flu, they are actually harmful.

So, the conclusion is: don't recommend treatments without good evidence in the form of a controlled trial. In 1938 a powerful, man-made oestrogen drug was created called diethylstilbestrol. It was widely advertised as Desplex for menopausal symptoms, *'morning after'* contraception and to prevent miscarriage. One advert, from 1957, said that it was *'recommended for routine prophylaxis in all pregnancies'* because it could *'prevent abortion, miscarriage and premature labour'* with *'96% live delivery with Desplex in one series of 1,200 patients – bigger and stronger babies too. No gastric or other side effects with Desplex – in either high or low dosage'.*[12]

The drug was originally introduced after it appeared that it was effective for stopping miscarriage.[13] However, there had been no control group – no comparator women by which we would know the difference that the drug made. By the time controlled trials were eventually reported in 1953 it was clear that the drug did not prevent miscarriages.[14] There was no advantage to the drug – but it had taken controlled trials to prove it. Worse, though, the drug increased the risk of vaginal cancer in the babies born to women who had taken it, along with an increased risk of breast cancer. When these babies grew up, their own pregnancies had an increased risk of premature birth and miscarriage.[15]

Desplex was a false promise with real harm – harm which was passed through the generations to the children of children exposed to it. This was and is outrageous. Harms will always happen in medicine, but this was an avoidable harm. It could have been foreseen had we asked: how do we know this works, beyond our mere opinion? And how do we know that it is not harmful?

In the 18th century James Lind had understood that effective treatments would only come about from paying attention to evidence, not opinion. Bennett spoke out in 1857 because he had reason to believe that unintended harm was occurring through inadequately tested interventions. We have just the same problems today. Medicine which does as little harm and as much good as possible relies on both sound science and people willing to speak up – often risking their own reputation, comfort or job security as they do so. There is an ongoing tension between the wish for innovation, improvement, the *'new'* and the modern on the one hand,

and the need to be careful, check *'facts'*, test fairly and have consideration for the fact that medicine can harm.

Systematic reviews and complete research

This book is not an argument that we should base every decision in healthcare on randomised controlled trials. It is, however, an argument that we need to pay much better attention to the need for evidence on where avoidable stresses on the NHS come from and how to ensure we spend money wisely. This means that we must ensure we know about gaps in evidence, are cognisant of the uncertainties that the current evidence contains and always consider the possibility of harm through our interventions.

If you are told that a new drug or treatment will improve the care of people with heart conditions because studies in rats have indicated that it might be useful, it is rational to consider a trial in human beings. Suppose a previous trial had shown the drug was ineffective – or, worse, it actually killed patients – you would want to make sure that what seemed at first to be a good idea was stopped from going ahead.

Clearly, it should be essential not to trial innovations without checking first whether they have been tried out before, and being attentive to the result. But in practice this checking is not routine: in popular medical journals researchers rarely stated they had systemically examined the research on the topic before they began.[16] The gold standard for checking the research terrain is known as a systematic review, a methodologically exacting search of what evidence is currently known. Unless this kind of review happens before the research starts, doctors with good intentions can kill patients.

In 2006, eight volunteers took part in a drug study, TGN1412, in Northwick Park Hospital in London. It should have been a straightforward experiment, but it ended up as a disaster. Six of the volunteers were injected with a monoclonal antibody, which it was hoped would be useful for people with conditions like leukaemia or rheumatoid arthritis. The other two had a placebo treatment. The six having the active treatment rapidly developed multiple organ failure.[17] Critically ill, they were all admitted to intensive care, the lungs, heart and kidneys requiring supportive care.[18] At least one of the trial volunteers had to have toes and fingers amputated.

The antibody hadn't been tested in humans before. Does this mean the harm was unpredictable? According to two researchers, analysing events in the *Lancet*, probably not. They described it as a *'high risk compound unlikely to be suitable for administration to healthy people without additional preclinical experiments'*. They argued that using the detail from animal and laboratory studies could have been used to better predict what would happen, and pertinent published work on the antibodies and antigens was not included in the pharmaceutical company's documentation. This meant that *'either possibility – activation or immunosuppression – could not be ruled out with the available data and, since these effects would have serious outcomes, the risk category should have been increased accordingly.'*[19]

In the trial, the volunteers' immune systems had been catastrophically activated. The humans, they argued, should only have been given a fraction of the dose the animals had received, yet the volunteers were given the same. Had this information been gathered and assessed, the hospitalisation and permanent damage to six people's health may have been avoided.

This was a dramatic harm attracting much media attention. Many others are neither as newsworthy or obvious. Certainly, some harms in medicine are hard – or impossible – to avoid. Others are far easier. Disregarding what is already known about a treatment or intervention, or failing to do basic tests first, should be unforgivable. Indeed, Iain Chalmers (who has worked tirelessly for better tests in healthcare) has written of how research continues to be done by companies blind to the fact that the same drugs have been tested by their competitors and found to be useless or harmful.[20]

It's clear that the TGN1412 trial should have had a systematic review of the knowledge on this monoclonal antibody, with adjustments made to the way the trial was run as a consequence of that knowledge. (Further human trials, with minute doses of the same drug, have continued and may still turn out to have value for some patients.[21]) A very similar problem occurred in the US in 2002 during a trial for an inhaled drug, hexamethonium, when a healthy volunteer died from lung failure several weeks after taking it. In fact, data showing that hexamethonium was toxic to humans was available from the 1950s, but this research was not contained in the computer search used, which dated back only to the mid-1960s.[22]

Equally, a lack of appreciation of the current knowledge in an area can mean that useful treatments don't get offered. A good example is the use of steroids to help mature the lungs of premature babies. A major cause of death in these tiny babies is lung disease, and trials started in the early 1970s to find out whether giving the mothers steroids just before birth would improve the premature babies' health. Indeed it did, and subsequent trials confirmed this. However, a systematic review was not published until 1989.[23] Use of steroids began to rise from 20% at the time of publication to 65% by 1996. Over the same period, death rates of premature babies fell. The effect of the delay in publishing a systematic review that made the benefits of steroids clear is, according to the Cochrane Collaboration: *'... tens of thousands of premature babies have probably suffered and died unnecessarily.'*

High-quality research, capable of answering the questions which are important to patients, families, carers and health professionals, is fundamental to providing good-quality healthcare. We have to be able to put aside our own biases in order to find out whether this will help or harm.

And that research needs to be complete. When the diligent look for evidence, they can only see what is there. Unpublished medical research[24] has been a scandal for decades. The AllTrials campaign[25] has rightfully drawn attention to such a nonsensical state of affairs: essentially, it is legal for drug companies to do a clinical trial, find that the drug under test does harm and then bury the results so that patients taking the medicines, and doctors prescribing the medicines, know nothing about it. In a series published in 2015, only 13.4% of trials had summary data published within one year.[26] This results in massive and unnecessary uncertainties.

In the UK, the antiviral medication oseltamivir, traded as Tamiflu, was stockpiled at a cost of £464 million to be used during a flu epidemic.[27] Is it useful in a flu epidemic? Does it prevent deaths or stop people from needing hospital care? Is it worth this expenditure? When the World Health Organisation (WHO) recommended its use, and the Centers for Disease Control and Prevention (CDC) in the US had recommended that it should be stockpiled in case of an epidemic, they had not seen the full trial data on the drug.[28] In the UK, the Medicines and Healthcare Products Regulatory Agency (MHRA) was sure it had all the relevant data when granting it a licence.[29] But it did not, and when the trial data was eventually obtained from Roche, the drug manufacturer, an independent systematic review concluded that the relatively minor improvement Tamiflu made came at the cost of side effects: *'Our results show that oseltamivir reduces the proportion of participants with symptomatic influenza when used for prophylaxis and has modest symptomatic effects when used for treatment, but it causes nausea and vomiting and increases the risk of headaches and renal and psychiatric syndromes.'* The researchers criticised governments intending to *'distribute oseltamivir to healthy people to prevent complications and interrupt transmission on the basis of a published evidence base that has been affected by reporting bias, ghost authorship, and poor methods'.*[30]

The Tamiflu purchased at great cost went out of date or was written off due to poor storage. What a waste, driven by systems that did not prioritise the need to publish all the relevant data for robust, critical, independent analysis of clinical trials. There was no refund: the money that could have been spent on things that we know work – like ensuring enough staff are available to look after patients – was gone.

Looking for harms

When we do not actively search for what is already known about a healthcare intervention, and we lack access to the raw data about it already generated, we do real and active damage, repeating mistakes that have already been made, unwittingly sacrificing time, money and potentially lives. When we do not prioritise finding out the harms of medicine, we do a disservice, because we either prescribe dangerous substances or we blindside people as to the true balance of benefit and harm. And when we are slow to admit our uncertainty or we do not publicly disclose harms as soon as we know about them, we screw up medicine for everyone. We have seen this recently in the enormous health checks scheme, a policy which the government mandated to all local health authorities. Yet there is high-quality evidence that these do not prevent death or illness, and instead may be directing even more resources at the most fit and well people.[31]

The same principles hold true for healthcare policy changes or innovations. We make a mess of our NHS by applying the same bad principles of chosen ignorance to swathes of clinical practice.

As we have seen, a recurrent theme of healthcare delivery has been its lack of attention to harm. This is not just something obvious, such as a surgeon who amputates the wrong leg or a nurse who gives penicillin to a patient known to be allergic to it. For example, side effects can occur because of the way healthcare systems are set up and organised; and they can occur with good intentions, and even through verbal or written communication.

Take a patient, let's call her Patricia, who has had a letter from her doctor urging her to make an appointment for a blood pressure check. She goes to the surgery reluctantly, where she is told her blood pressure is slightly raised. But the nurse, Beth, then asks her to step on the weighing scales. Patricia had not expected this. She knows she is overweight and feels humiliated. She only came for a blood pressure check. She wishes she hadn't come. The nurse tells her, *'You are very overweight; your body mass index is 35, and you are running a big risk of a heart attack or stroke'.* Patricia puts on her jacket and leaves, saying thank you, but feeling angry at what has happened.

From the nurse's point of view, she has done a useful thing. Beth has read a recent report about the impact of obesity in society, and a research paper stating that primary care staff should do more to prevent this *'timebomb'.* She feels that, as the research says,[32] the patient was probably unaware that she was overweight, and she has therefore given Patricia useful information, and would have talked more, given more time. Beth has done what she has been told to do. She has brought up the subject of weight, as the National Obesity Forum has recommended.[33] It says that staff should make every contact with patients count: *'Very few patients will cite obesity or weight management as the reason for seeing their GP, and will instead present with conditions that are clearly a result of weight issues. GPs should talk with their patients about weight in these instances.'* Beth has transgressed the *'barriers'* to discussing weight with a patient, demonstrating her wish to change her patients behaviour, as recommended by other researchers.[34]

But does the evidence actually say that healthcare professionals asking about weight will be useful? Despite the policy generated by politicians, pushed for by charities and endorsed by the media at large, there is a lack of evidence proving that professionals telling patients to lose weight results in medium or long-term benefits,[35] and even the commercial weight-loss programmes, which many GPs can now refer to, are not useful for most: as we have seen, only ten people in every 1,000 to whom they are recommended will end up with long-term weight loss.[36] And what are the harms of GPs asking people to lose weight? What damage could the motivated, kind Beth have done? As one patient says: *'Almost every consultation I've ever had – about glandular fever, contraception, a sprained ankle – has included a conversation about my weight; and that's inevitably the conversation that destroys any rapport or trust that might have existed between me and my doctor.'* [37]

The reasons as to why Patricia is overweight are complex, a complex interlacing series of issues to do with being made redundant, the death of her husband ten years ago, the debt she is now in, the low mood that persists despite the appointment at a counsellor, and her lack of social or food networks locally. Her weight continues to increase over the coming months and years. She feels guilt, sadness and a loss of control.

And here is a rare study of harm that is relevant: when people perceive themselves to be overweight, they are more likely to gain rather than lose weight over the coming years.[38] Beth's intervention may potentially have exacerbated Patricia's weight problem. A few years later, Patricia finds a lump in her breast. She knows that she should see someone about this, but she recalls her last visit to her general practice and feels shame. She thinks she will be told, if it's cancer, that it's her fault; she's too fat. She puts off making the appointment again and again. And this is another harm.

This bad outcome is a subtle one. It was caused originally by good intentions in a pressured system. We would be unlikely to know why Patricia delayed going to her doctor unless we considered that a seemingly helpful comment was potentially harmful. Even then, looking for that harm as part of a research project would have to be done very carefully. This lack of investigation of harm in medicine is endemic. Screening (testing well people in order to find early signs of disease) can often do harm. This harm is mainly through finding abnormalities that would never have led to health problems in the future, meaning that the person gets side effects from the treatment but no hope of benefit from it (overtreatment) and false positive findings (when the test appears to show a problem when there is, in fact, no abnormality).

It would seem to be obvious, then, that trials investigating screening should ensure they look for harms and not just benefits. Yet an analysis of 198 trials of screening found that in only a minority of instances were the harms outlined – just 7% quantified overdiagnosis (finding abnormalities which would never go on to create problems) and 4% quantified false positive findings.[39] This means that a massive portion of research is unbalanced – it is unable to inform us fairly about the downsides of screening. How can we create a sustainable NHS when we don't examine whether the money we spend is doing more harm than good?

'Opportunity costs'

Let us imagine the NHS as a large cake. If the cake size stays the same, the only way to divide it out into more *'slices'*, is for many people to get less. Every time there is a new policy initiative, as well as asking myself whether this will work and is it better for patients? I want to know: if we are not making a bigger cake, then what do we have to stop doing in order to fit this in instead? Otherwise, many people will be left with unsatisfying crumbs.

This dilemma is known in microeconomics as *'opportunity costs'*. Stopping the NHS from doing things that don't work would be rational, sensible and efficient. Not starting new things that will not work would be even more logical, because it would prevent us from losing money and time unnecessarily.

Let's take as an example the prescribing of statins. NICE made the decision in 2015 to prescribe them to people whose projected risk of heart attack or stroke in the next ten years – based on factors like blood pressure, cholesterol, family history or smoking – was 10%.[40] NICE changed it from 20% on the basis of a cost-effectiveness calculation: essentially, the cost of the statins (tumbling in price thanks to generic manufacture) is less than the cost of treating the heart attacks and strokes that NICE calculated would otherwise occur. But what NICE didn't factor was the impact of providing more GP appointments: to have a discussion about whether or not they wanted their risk to be calculated, to have the necessary measurements taken and calculated, and then to have a follow-up discussion about whether or not a statin was wanted. Indeed, what may look like a simple discussion may be multifaceted: a friend or relative may be on statins whose experience has been noted, for good or bad; there may be a desire not to take more tablets, no matter what their risk calculation says; or perhaps the patient's father had an early heart attack and dreads their own level of risk being revealed.

Incredibly, NICE stated that it *'does not believe the new guidance will increase workload for GPs'*.[41] What parallel universe is this, where it will take no more time for GPs to assess, discuss, monitor or treat 4.5 million people? In fact, NICE's own evidence review reported that: *'Expert opinion suggests that there is insufficient capacity within existing primary care resources to meet the increase in demand as a result of implementing the guideline.'*[42] With no mechanism to formally investigate opportunity cost, how would NICE have known?

Instead, the resultant harms from such a policy go unseen and uncounted: the man who wanted to talk about his suicidal thoughts but can't get an appointment this week because the general practice has had to use those appointments for people to discuss their cholesterol; or the GP who becomes stressed at the impossibility of doing a good enough job, slides into burnout and depression, resigns and can't be replaced, leaving even fewer appointments for people who want them. Stressed systems are poorly operating systems and incur avoidable harms. So when organisations make policy recommendations without investigating opportunity costs, we have no idea whether, overall, we are doing more good than harm.

Another example is the health secretary's idea[43] to print the cost of drugs onto prescriptions when they are more than £20, in order to *'reduce waste by reminding people of the cost of medicine, but also improve patient care by boosting adherence to drug regimes'*. There is no evidence this is the case. There are numerous possible harms: people feel too guilty to reorder their medicines; people feel shame, embarrassment or fear. It would be entirely possible to run a trial to find out what is most useful and least harmful. (And what about the people who pay the full prescription charge for medications that cost pennies – will they be told and feel resentful that they are subsidising cost to others?)

Jeremy Hunt also proposed that people be told how much a missed appointment cost the NHS.[44] In this case there was a trial – good – which showed that text-messaging reminders about appointments that included a note about the cost to the NHS resulted in a reduction in missed appointments.[45] However, the only measures were of whether people went to the appointment or not: there was no evaluation of any harms, or assessment of what patients thought about it.[46] One of my tasks as a GP is to persuade people that their needs are great enough to merit treatment. A common statement from older people is *not worth it at my age*. What would the impact have been – would people be more likely to take or stop medication, or feel guilt? What would Patricia have made of it? But there was no mention of testing out this idea in a trial, which would have been straightforward to do and learn from.

The NHS has always had high intrinsic moral value. Its purpose is to treat suffering, based on need, regardless of the individual's ability to pay, race, gender or religion, and aspiring to the highest standards of professionalism and excellence as it does so.[47] But good intentions are not enough. The NHS constitution also states: *The NHS is committed to providing best value for taxpayers' money and the most effective, fair and sustainable use of finite resources.* In other words, don't waste money and spend time wisely. Searching for the most effective ways to do things would mean that we ensured we looked at all the evidence before we began to use a new intervention. It would mean testing them fairly, and searching for harms and considering opportunity costs. It would ensure that we were doing things that mattered to patients and their families, not just to politicians.

So what happens when politicians develop health interventions based on political philosophy and without full regard for the evidence? The next chapter examines the NHS's recent history when it has done exactly that.

Interview

Kenneth Arrow, professor of economics and Nobel Prize winner

When you are buying medical help for illness, it's rather different from buying food. It's sporadic, unpredictable. It's a random event. There's a lot of uncertainty; the cost can be rather large, and the value can be rather great. The need for healthcare only comes in a variable and uncertain way.

In the modern world, there are three elements to the healthcare story. From a US point of view, the triad is patient, physician and insurer. The insurance part is not that old – I can remember a point where hospital insurance was new, and insurance was for hospital care only. I can remember a physician friend of mine telling me in the immediate post-war (World War II, that is) period that there were a couple of companies offering outpatient insurance, but it was very inadequate then – just for unionised working men, for example. In a few years we had a bigger spread of offerings by private insurance companies and also by co-operatives, who played a pioneering but transitory role. So: you want good care, and the financial costs are high. In many fields, you do have insurance – but for, say, house insurance, it's for an event that is easily identifiable and where the costs of repair are not very uncertain. For example, a house burns down. You experience damages which can be remedied at a fairly well-known cost. With illness, you have a new factor, a physician – and many other healthcare professionals. There's no equivalent in most other forms of insurance. We are now dealing with this trinity, this trio – patient, insurer, doctor. Being a physician means having certain kinds of knowledge – that's why you go to the physician; he or she knows better than you do, and as a result, you can't really check on how well they have done. When I buy a car, I can't make it, but I can check its performance easily. I can test drive it, I can read descriptions, I can know if it's reliable. But if I 'buy' a physician, I really don't know if I'm missing something important. The physician might not be as well trained as I think. There is a consequence. The usual argument for a good market is that you depend on both sides of the market being well informed as to the quality of what's on sale. But that doesn't apply here.

The second problem is between the insurer and the physician. The insurer may be better informed than the patient. But the insurer can't really check what the physician is doing. The insurer does not know, or can't keep track of that – it would be too much interference if they did. So you have this 'drop out'. When markets work well, it's when both sides are reasonably well informed as to the quality of the product and the financial terms. You assume there is a price at which you can choose to buy or not buy. You at least know what you are getting. However, there are three parties here, and each has varying degrees of information about each other. Further, the stakes are high. It's not as though it is a small matter. If I get a car repaired, it may be true that I don't know much about repairs and that the repairer may cheat me. It's similar to healthcare, but the stakes are much lower. But here, in healthcare, it can be extremely serious. Now, the system problem is exacerbated by the fact that medical practice is a good deal better than it used to be – all sorts of things can be done where they couldn't before. But by the same token, differences in information – among patients, physicians, insurers – have become greater. As a result, the costs and the effects on the economy are much higher. The conclusion is that ordinary markets are inadequate.

What would happen if you had more information about performance? We in the United States have this very complicated system – it's chaotic – and we are getting more performance information. It applies more to hospitals than physicians in general. There are ratings of hospitals, providers. You get hospitals who look worse. And they say, well, we take the hard cases. And it's frequently true. It's a real issue, a real difficulty. People who take the hard cases are going to look less good.

You ask whether this kind of information – rating systems and so forth – will ever get good enough to rely on and thus make a normal 'health market' achievable?' I think the answer is, no. There is a tendency to inform the patient more and allow him or her to make more decisions, but this is in the course of treatment, well after the point at which markets would be relevant. When the individual signs up for an insurance policy or health plan, he or she can hardly anticipate all the choices which will have to be made.

What was the reaction to my paper ('Uncertainty and the Welfare Economics of Medical Care', 1963)? Well, I'm not a policymaker. I was just saying, the market isn't good, here – you can't just leave [healthcare] to the market. I did establish that case. If anything came out of it, it was about the code of ethics, the way that doctors police each other. How do you establish codes of conduct that people believe in? Well, something Americans go in for, far more than the British, is litigation. So the kind of evidence that comes on board is, 'what this doctor did was not in keeping with the standards.' These ethical codes actually wind up as a legal act. It's a fairly roundabout method, and it costs.

The best system here seems to be where you combine insurance with healthcare (the so-called health maintenance organisation) – a company that provides both, like Kaiser Permanente. Covering healthcare with insurance was originally linked to employment – which is a strange thing. They are quite different realms. Health insurance plans came in during World War II as part of the competition for labour, and a lot did give family coverage, but of course there were gaps – women were less significant in the labour force at that time. Now, we have some universal coverage – like Medicare for retired people. Even that's been under attack. Leading Republicans have suggested that, instead of reimbursements, you give vouchers, and you can buy any insurance policy you want. It's a dangerous step. Individuals are a poor judge of appropriate insurance policies, because they are too complicated. There is such a variety of medical possibilities and it's very hard to comparison-shop amongst policies. We are doing this more with Obamacare – the Affordable Care Act – where people of working age can buy private insurance, with a subsidy if income is low. But you still have to choose an insurance policy. There is some provision to make it easier to make comparisons, but it's clear that many people are buying policies poorly – it's very hard to make these decisions.

In practice, the theoretical advantages of choice are outweighed by the fact that people don't do a good job of making these choices in a competitive environment – it's almost impossible. The evidence here is that people make poor choices, and the choices are often not very good. The best-value systems are where insurance and provision are combined – like Kaiser. But they have not grown or expanded into other parts of the country. The National Health Service is a similar idea. The normal market system does include people going out of business if that business turns out to be inefficient, if you misguess your market, or if you misguess your costs. I live in Silicon Valley where there are loads of startups – and at least half of them fail. That's normal; it's part of a competitive system. It's a problem if it happens in a medical system, because it interrupts care, and it's deleterious to an ongoing relationship; it's bad for people who were getting that service. But the fact that they fail is the way the market system works. Next time around, they'll guess their costs better. But if you are right in the middle of medical care and the supplier goes broke, you have adjustment costs. It's not the same if I'm buying fruit and they go out of business – well, I can go to a nearby store.

Medical markets are just different. They are not the same as buying fruit. Some of us here do use the NHS as a good example of healthcare – the longevity of people is better, the costs are very much lower. Our longevity here in the US is lower than that in Cuba! The NHS has stood out as a cost-effective system achieving a good health standard. I'm so surprised that a country that has contained its costs and achieved good healthcare should be worried.

5

The Political NHS

The NHS, as Bevan recognised, has to operate within a budget. It will never be able to work without limits. We can debate what that budget might be, and how much of our Gross Domestic Product (GDP) should be used to fund the NHS, but it will always be finite. The NHS could spend infinite amounts on healthcare – more staff, more research, better hospitals, new treatments for cancer, searching for genetic risk factors, treating infertility, funding pharmaceuticals for dementia. If we don't want to waste precious financial resources, we have to ask what spending gives us value for money and what does not?

One challenge is that political promises do not always get kept. For example, in 2009 David Cameron said, *'with the Conservatives there will be no more of the tiresome, meddlesome, top-down re-structures that have dominated the last decade of the NHS'.*[1] This declaration was followed, in 2012, by the Health and Social Care Act, which was, according to the then Chief Executive of the NHS, *'big enough to be seen from space'.*[2] A second problem is asking voters to make choices based on poor information, which is compounded by the perpetual temptation of making decisions based on our own prejudices, or, as we have seen, on the basis of underexplained information or a lack of data on potential harms.

There are many routes through which the activities of the NHS are directed, but the ruling government has ultimate control. Our politicians are able to make powerful decisions about how the NHS is run, which they often – but not always – declare in their election manifestos. In 2015 the Conservatives promised a *'7-day NHS'*. In a democracy, isn't it a good idea to elect the party who will apportion spending to what the people want – better care for people with dementia, or more resources to deal with people with learning difficulties – why should that be a problem? Politicians in the last few decades have sought increasing control over doctors – especially GPs, who have found their consultations increasingly micromanaged. In the belief that financial rewards result in better medical care, politicians have incentivised doctors' activities by directly linking payments to outcomes by creating a target culture. A similar belief that more competition will lead to higher standards has resulted in the increased use of data to judge and compare services. But these developments have ignored the issues of opportunity costs, resulted in perverse outcomes and have given little benefit to patients while wasting resources. The lessons from evidence-based medicine have been ignored.

The *'7-day NHS'*

So, when the Conservatives pledged in their 2015 manifesto to provide '*7-day a week access to your GP and deliver a truly 7-day NHS*',[3] how many people stopped to ask what this meant, whether it was worth the money or what the harms might be? In truth, when I read it before the election, I didn't give it a second thought. We already have an NHS working seven days a week, I thought: this is a promise that doesn't need any actions.

NHS services have always been organised to take account of emergency care. Staff have always worked in rota systems at weekends, overnights, high days and holidays. There are undoubtedly less staff on at weekends compared to weekdays, because staff at weekends are there to deal with urgent and emergency care, whether in general practice or in hospitals, while routine work is done during the week – be it hip replacements, cataract surgery, outpatient clinic visits, meetings to discuss the ongoing care of people with mental illness, meetings to plan the future organisational changes needed in services, cervical screening, routine blood test monitoring for people with chronic illness, and so on. This means that more staff are naturally needed during the routine working hours – usually 8 a.m. to 6 p.m., slightly longer in general practice. Additionally, where problems in accessing services have been identified – for example, in stroke care – specific units have been created that have ensured patients have access to tests, investigations and staff,[4] but this provision all happened without any political involvement.

It is, of course, reasonable to argue that routine care should be available at weekends as well as weekdays. Patients work, often having caring responsibilities and busy lives. However, it costs to provide and requires major redistribution of resources. Junior doctors, who work 48-hour weeks,[5] have always been paid more for *'unsocial'* hours. Consultants have a different scheme whereby they are paid in relation to how many hours they work in daytime hours added to on call pay. This pay is related to the intensity of their out-of-daytime-hours jobs – so doctors who are spending most of their time in the hospital overnight or at weekends will get paid more compared to consultants who rarely need to come in. Therefore, the problem with shifting more routine work to weekends is not just the need to pay staff more to work unsocial hours.

The government's proposals, set out by Jeremy Hunt, resulted in an outpouring of medical opposition united by two things: evidence and attitude. Hunt had claimed that there was a need for a new contract *'that brings back a sense of vocation'*, and that medicine had become *'a Monday to Friday profession'* where *'you end up with catastrophic consequences'*. He told the BBC that the previous Labour administration had allowed consultants to opt out of weekends on call, and *'now, if you are admitted on a Sunday, you are 15% more likely to die than if you are admitted on a Wednesday, and we have about 6,000 avoidable deaths each year'*. He ended by saying, *'What is causing those deaths? Lack of senior consultant cover at weekends is one of the critical points'.*[6] In November 2015, the contract issues between junior doctors (that is, any doctor not a fully qualified GP or consultant : the word *'junior'* belies the fact that these doctors are often highly experienced, making high-level, critical decisions) and the government became a major dispute when 98% of junior doctors voted for strike action.[7] Critically, senior consultants stood behind them in full vocal support,[8] as did GPs.[9]

Part of Hunt's proposal to junior doctors, which had precipitated the vote, was to make more hours paid as 'routine' at the weekend or up to 10 p.m. at night, but it was his comments that lit the blue touchpaper. A social media campaign started with doctors (along with many other healthcare professionals) posting photos of themselves at work on weekends, along with the hashtag (the twitter indexing system) #iminworkjeremy. A palpable outpouring of anger greeted the assertion that doctors were no longer acting out of vocation.

In fact, a slow burn staff shortage across medicine had now reached boiling point. In the 2010s, a cumulative staffing crisis in general practice meant that in some areas, a quarter of evening and weekend shifts were going unfilled – and this is core cover for urgent and emergency care.[10] Similarly, in hospitals, enormous sums of money were being paid to attract locum doctors to fill emergency shifts – the NHS was expected to spend 3.7 billion on agency staff in NHS hospitals in 2015/16[11] to keep such unfilled shifts afloat. With 80% of Trusts in the red in 2014/15, this meant huge, bankrupting, sums of money being spent to ensure a minimum of staff for urgent and emergency care alone.[12] There were too few doctors available to work these core shifts. How could extending routine work to weekends be possible, never mind affordable?

In primary care, the situation had similarities and differences. Urgent care at weekends, evenings and nights had mainly been hived off to out-of-hours centres during the 1990s. By the 2010s, the government started to offer GPs money to open up for more routine appointments either early in the morning, in the evenings or on Saturday mornings.[13] From 2013, pilots extended the scheme in England, at a cost of £150 million,[14] and the Department of Health stated that the intention was to roll it out across all GP surgeries by

2020.[15] Was this worth the money? Over 800,000 people were surveyed and more than 80% had no problem with their GP opening hours, and while Saturday access would suit some, Sunday was less popular.[16] In any event, some areas stopped the schemes after the hoped-for reduction in A&E attendances didn't happen, finding that the schemes just increased costs.[17] By late 2015, half of pilot sites had stopped or cut back some or all of their added hours because they were either unpopular or underused.[18]

In other words, offering a seven-day-a-week GP service was a political confection. Most people didn't have a problem with accessing care during normal opening hours, and Sundays in particular were wasting money through underuse. Yet, rather than looking to add extra services, the NHS was already under enormous pressure maintaining the core service of urgent and emergency care seven days a week, 24 hours a day. As the Nuffield Trust put it: *'Services that seek only to extend access to general practice across longer hours may end up resolving clinical problems and generating additional demand in approximately equal measure and at high cost.'*[19] And, like everything in medicine, changing policy can create other harms. General practices were already in a state of meltdown, with many practices in a funding crisis, unable to recruit enough doctors, facing closures.[20] Spreading doctors even more thinly risks disrupting continuity, where you can no longer see the same doctor most of the time – meaning that patients have to repeat themselves every time. Continuity is also associated with higher quality of care and lower costs.[21] GPs who might have worked in urgent and emergency services may end up working additional evening or weekend routine hours instead, making urgent services even less well staffed. Yet none of these harms were examined when the policy was being pushed through.

The *'7-day NHS'*, as defined by the Conservatives, was a highly political policy, expected to have popular – though superficial – appeal. It did not take account of what was currently happening, what the needs of the population were or where it might be wasteful if their vision were implemented. Unintended consequences – not least funding shortfalls, opportunity costs, and less continuity of care – were not accounted for.

Hunt was challenged, repeatedly, on his interpretation of the statistics around weekends in the NHS. He made two big mistakes: he confused association with causation and he made an inference as to the cause. The first is an elementary error; in my house it's called the *'yellow socks'* issue. Some time ago, my youngest child was learning how to do handstands, tutored by an older sibling. The following day, he couldn't manage a rerun of his feat. He ran upstairs. What's the matter? I called. I've gone to get my yellow socks, he said. I had them on yesterday – I'll put them on and that'll fix the problem. It was a perfect, but perfectly wrong explanation and action. Yellow socks did not make my youngest able to do handstands. But it was associated with his ability to do handstands because the day that he got the most coaching, help and support to do it, he was wearing them. It was not the socks, but the sister assisting him that made the difference.

Hunt is not the only person to have confused association and causation. This phenomenon bedevils many 'big data' papers, where large datasets are used to observe NHS activity but cannot explain them. In Hunt's case, the data was deaths related to the day the patient was admitted to hospital. These kinds of results – observational data – are often very interesting and useful, but they cannot reliably determine what is cause and what is effect; that usually needs randomised controlled trials.

Hunt took the observational data on weekend death rates and then stated that a large part of the cause was a lack of consultants at weekends, and he would not back down from his assertion: *'I cannot negotiate about a promise we made in a manifesto. I have an obligation to deliver that manifesto.'*[22] Not only did he personalise the problem with a suggestion that consultants did not work weekends but he also missed the point. During the week, people are admitted to hospital for tests or procedures as a *'routine'* case – by definition, they are less sick than people admitted as an emergency; there is a bigger proportion of emergencies at the weekend, when people who can be dealt with as *'routine'* are not normally admitted. These crucial adjustments had been partially or completely missing from the initial papers on weekend working. Other researchers have found an increase in deaths following hip fractures in patients admitted at the weekend – even with a consultant-led service every day of the week.[23] Hunt had said that there were *'6,000 avoidable deaths a year'* – but whether they were avoidable was entirely unproven.[24] Are the factors which cause people to be admitted at the weekend rather than through the week (perhaps alcohol or travel, or a lack of social services) associated with different kinds of people with different risk factors? In fact, even the research paper itself[25] made clear that, *'it is not possible to ascertain the extent to which these excess deaths may be preventable; to assume that they are avoidable would be rash and misleading'*. And, indeed, another paper published in 2016 found that people being admitted at the weekend were sicker compared to people being admitted during the week.[26] Instead of a well-informed, fundamental debate about what meaning could be attached to the numbers and how the NHS should best address it, the issue became a nasty, personalised fight. Much the same could be said for many of the tranches of big data that are produced in healthcare.

Clearly, if there were evidence of delays in providing emergency care at different times of the day or night that would indicate that services should be reorganised. But it would be a mistake to think that this is all about doctors. An emergency coronary angiography requires not just a doctor but specialist nurses, cardiac technicians, porters, radiographers and laboratory staff to run the blood tests that need to be done. In the daytime, there is more flexibility if a sudden surge in emergencies occurs – staff who are present to do routine work can cancel that and work on the emergency side instead. (This happens constantly. It is one of the reasons why thousands of operations are cancelled every year.) A change to identical services every day of the week would cost not just doctors' salaries, but many others too.

Hunt's plan, though, was not just to have more doctors rostered for weekends, it also appeared to be about shifting more routine work to weekends – in both primary and secondary care. With less staff present on any weekday as they get thinned out to an even spread across seven days – there would be a cost of over a billion pounds and side effects other than simply where the money is taken from. As some health economists have put it: *'There is as yet no clear evidence that 7-day services will reduce weekend deaths or can be achieved without increasing weekday deaths. The planned cost of implementing 7-day services greatly exceeds the maximum amount that the National Health Service should spend on eradicating the weekend effect based on current evidence.'*[27] Hunt later appeared to backtrack, saying that his focus was on emergency and urgent care: this was clearly not the case for general practice.[28]

The problem with misunderstanding statistics is that we end up offering the wrong solution to a complex set of data. There may be a problem with the way the NHS organises its services over the days, and there may be ways that we can and should do better. But the data Hunt used was not designed or able to answer these questions. Data about weekends and death rates is observational – it is full of questions, uncertainties, the unexplained and the unexpected. None of this means that there is not a problem with weekend care – the data Hunt cited could not prove this – and none of this means that the NHS could not do better. But Hunt did a silly thing, which was to purport to find evidence that enhanced, retrospectively, his political policy. This political policy as the *'solution'* to it is misguided, because it risks taking money from places where it is working and putting it in places where it won't help. The government had an opportunity to ask for expert help in interpreting the data, working out what it meant and matching it to what was already known – instead, the National

Statistics Authority rebutted the secretary of state's claims. The *weekend effect* (higher mortality at the weekend) has been found in several developed countries[29] and that the cause, or how to mitigate it, is not known.[30] To add insult to injury, Hunt also claimed that *currently, across all key specialties, in only 10% of our hospitals are patients seen by a consultant within 14 hours of being admitted at the weekend*,[31] which is incorrect. As Dr David Craven, a Royal Society Research fellow put it, it was *simply impossible* to conclude this from the data, which didn't separate out weekend and weekdays.[32] To paraphrase American journalist H.L. Mencken: For every complex problem – such as how best to organise medical staffing at weekends in the NHS – there is an answer that is clear, simple and wrong. This issue needs unbiased minds and clear statistical understanding – not an election manifesto promise to be driven through no matter the cost. The cost of this political nonsense was to anger doctors and confuse the public: doctors started to note the *'Hunt effect'* when ill patients asked not to be admitted to hospital at the weekend and wait till Monday instead. Truly, unless we actively look for harms we shall never find them.

Payments, outcomes and warped incentives

The GP contract of 2004 was a revolution in how GPs were paid. Until then, payments were made for tasks, such as prescribing contraception, providing vaccinations and smear tests. After most medical records had moved onto computer it meant new tranches of data were available at a click. A couple of decades ago, if I wanted to know how many people in the practice has asthma, I would have to ask the practice manager. She would have a list. This list would have been generated by doctors giving her, over the last weeks, months and years, a bit of paper on which the patient's name and diagnosis had been written. She would have added the name and date of birth to another bit of paper in a ring binder, which at some point became a computer record. It's easy to see the problems: doctors forget to add patients on, there are time delays, patients move away, bits of paper get easily lost in a busy practice and among countless other bits of paper.

Computers made it possible to instantly add patients on to 'disease registers', which in turn meant that it was simple to arrange to send appointments for regular reviews. It was possible to check medications that people were on, ensuring they were up to date and correct according to the latest evidence. To start with, the GP contract focused on having registers of people with various conditions, such as learning disability or heart disease. This was quite useful because it ensured we knew which patients had what conditions, and it enabled good recall systems to monitor and update people's care. But over time the contract became more detailed and exacting. The computer was used to trigger questions about depression among people with chronic illness, to take down details of a patient's family history of heart disease, or ask and score how much exercise was being done.

Two reasons were given for recording increasing volumes of information. The first was to improve quality of care. The second was to pay per performance – for many of the boxes asking to be ticked were part of the growing tentacles of the GP contract. Did attaching payment to entering more data on the computer result in better outcomes for patients? And what were the harms of doing so? Shamefully, these questions are only starting to be answered, more than a decade after the new policies were introduced.

One recent target was for GPs making a diagnosis of dementia. The UK National Screening Committee (UKNSC) is an evidence-based organisation in charge of scrutinising the evidence relating to screening – that is, in testing people who are apparently well and show no signs or symptoms of illness. The UKNSC has consistently stated that screening people for dementia should not be done, because the harms outweigh the benefit. So, people with symptoms – or whose families or carers report possible symptoms – should be investigated for possible dementia, but people without symptoms should not be routinely screened. Not only are the tests ineffective, giving false positives almost a quarter of the time, but they miss about one-third of people with dementia as well.[33] This poor-quality test is therefore capable of doing harm.

In fact, diagnosing dementia is often extremely complex. The more subtle the symptoms and the earlier the diagnosis is made, the more uncertain it is. As we get older, memory changes and, for some people, it isn't as good. A variety of labels have been used to describe this, from *'benign senescent forgetfulness'* in the 1960s, to *'late life forgetfulness'* in the 1980s and the current *'mild cognitive impairment'*.[34] Crucially, however, these minor memory difficulties are not dementia. Dementia can only be diagnosed, by definition, when there is an ongoing functional impairment – *'an impact on daily functioning related to a decline in the ability to judge, think, plan and organise. There is an associated change in behaviour such as emotional lability, irritability, apathy or coarsening of social skills. There must be evidence of decline over time (months or years rather than days or weeks) to make a diagnosis of dementia.'* [35]

So common woes like not finishing the crossword quickly, or going into a living room and forgetting where you left the remote control are blips in memory rather than dementia. Nor is it a *'spot'* diagnosis. The only times I've been pretty sure on first discussion are when, say, a son or daughter brings a parent with a clear story of weeks or months of deteriorating abilities and their parent, on discussion, is confused, unable to remember things for short periods of time, and scores low on one of the standardised memory questionnaires. More commonly, someone has intermittent or mild problems with memory, dressing or shopping. Often there might well be an issue but it isn't interfering much with independent life. In these situations it is often a question of watching and waiting to see what will happen, while ensuring that there isn't any treatable cause (like medication) or risk factors that could be reduced (like smoking).

However, here comes the politics. The UK government decided that dementia wasn't being diagnosed often enough.

Alzheimer's charities agreed.[36] Hunt told the House of Commons that the rate of diagnosing dementia was *shockingly low*. This was based on statistics suggesting that just under half of patients with dementia were diagnosed with it.[37] New targets of increased diagnosis rates were set for GPs – with a new reward of £55 per patient for doing so.[38] GPs were told to ask their older patients if they were worried about their memory and, if so, to set up memory testing for them. Simon Stevens, chief executive of the NHS told the BBC that *'There are about 700,000 people who have probably got dementia across England, and at the moment just over half of those people who want to find out about that are [diagnosed].'* [39] – but without asking them, how would he know?

Was this a good idea? The government based its opinion on data from Delphi studies,[40] which are essentially expert reviews and consensus of the available literature. In the words of the report: *'Delphi consensus is a useful method for making estimates where an evidence base exists but data are incomplete, scanty or otherwise imperfect.'*

In the US, diagnostic codes are extremely important because they could trigger insurance payments for people who have been treated. In the UK, coding by GPs is mainly done for two reasons: payment and to help with summaries of past medical history. Practices are paid to keep up-to-date records of how many people need vaccinations or who have had heart attacks, for example. I might code *'back pain'* for one patient who has serious and recurrent bouts of debilitating pain. I probably won't for someone who mentions a back pain that lasted a few days and has now gone. Why? Functionality. If I have ten minutes with a patient I've never met before, I need a quick clean summary of their past medical history. Cluttering this with every symptom the patient has ever had means a list that's impossibly long to get a fast handle on significant conditions. As important is the issue of permanence. It is possible to remove a diagnostic code from notes, but requires time and justification to do. There is a trace left that may be of note to insurance companies and other parts of the healthcare service.

Personally I do not code where there is a moderate degree of uncertainty about the diagnosis. I am worried that by being too certain, I am giving a misleading sense of security about a memory symptom that could mean depression, drug effects or stress. With the diagnosis also comes prognosis. Dementia is organ failure – brain failure. In many ways it is a terminal illness. That has implications for the way investigations and treatments will be offered to that person for the rest of their life. A person with dementia is unlikely to benefit from aggressive treatment for cancer, because the dementia may well cause death first. All that is likely to happen is that the person would suffer more. However, a person whose memory problems were caused by depression would be expected to make a good recovery from the depression and should, if appropriate, have the aggressive cancer treated to try and cure it. The diagnosis shapes much about the future. And, finally, this is about honesty. Patients can rightly see everything that is written in their notes. This will naturally include all the diagnostic codes. I would not code anything in the records that the person didn't know about. Sharing uncertainty is what doctors do; but time itself is used as a diagnostic test. Persistent symptoms are far more likely to be significant than minor, intermittent or improving complaints. As the dementia 'Tsar', Professor Alisdair Burns, has co-written, '*It may not be possible to diagnose dementia in a single consultation but rather after a period of current and historic review of the patient*'.[41] If we are going to give bad news, we should at least be reasonably certain that it is correct news.

This is the complex jungle of symptoms, worry and uncertainty into which was entered a £55 bounty with the intention of raising the level of diagnosis to the 'correct' level, as predicted by the Delphi consensus.[42] Knowing how many people there are with dementia in your community is very useful to work out the number of social carers you need or nursing homes you need to build. However, the Delphi numbers weren't being used to work out the needs across a large population, but the diagnosis rates in small groups. If a practice looks after patients in three nursing homes, we would expect more people to have dementia than in a practice that mainly looks after university students. The studies analysed to create estimates reached different conclusions about the amount of people that would be expected to have dementia: for example, for people between the ages of 85–89, the rate of dementia varied between 16.1%, 20.7% and 25.4%. For a practice population of 100 in this age group, a doctor would expect – by the range of studies used – to have between 16 and 26 patients with dementia on the list. That's a large range of potentially 'correct' numbers. The Delphi estimate in 2014 concluded that 7.1% of people aged over 65 had dementia.[43] Normally, when research numbers are presented like this there is a 'confidence interval' expressed; for example, it could be '7.2% with 95% confidence that the true figure lies between 8% and 14%'. In other words, we can't be sure of the exact number, but we can be pretty sure that the answer lies between two estimates. However, there was no confidence interval. The researchers were clear that the result was an estimate with important uncertainties: 'there are important weaknesses', they wrote, for the data is 'dependent on the validity and generalisability of the available evidence'.

One would therefore expect a bit of caution in how the data was used in real life, but the government chose to publish 'dementia maps' that plotted the estimated numbers of people with dementia relative to the number of codes GPs had made in the records. This was reported in the press as 'best and worst' areas.[44] GPs were then told by the Department of Health what numbers of people with dementia they should expect, which led to GP Martin Brunet describing how:

'My own practice was given a diagnosis rate of 127% in 2013, which was then changed to 59% in 2014! To accurately estimate the number of cases in my practice would require a much more local form of measurement – something that takes into account not only age, but factors such as ethnic mix, the type of housing available, the number of nursing homes and whether or not homes specialise in dementia care.'

This level of care with the expected numbers of people with dementia wasn't done. Brunet illuminates the saga by comparing the margin of error provided for people with diabetes:

'For Surrey in 2014, for instance, the prevalence is estimated at 6.9%, with a possible range of 5–10%. This means a 5% margin for error, which is nearly as great as the figure itself – something that should ring alarm bells. Applied to my own practice our quoted diagnosis rate of 79% could actually be anywhere between 55% and 110%.' [45]

However, some GP managers told doctors that they should be able to find an extra 15 people with dementia per 2,000 patients on their list – an extraordinarily precise number – with accompanying cash payments.[46] How would patients feel if they knew that their doctor was asking these questions by rote for the cash?

So what, you may think, it's impossible to be accurate. Surely the point is that GPs weren't diagnosing dementia often enough and needed incentives to raise the bar? Isn't the greater harm not diagnosing people? We will never know the balance of benefit and harm that took place before the scheme was eventually withdrawn. GPs complained that patients hated being asked about their memory when they wanted to spend their limited time with the doctor on something more pressing.[47] What damage was done to the relationship between patient and doctor? Do doctors deserve to be trusted if they ask questions which are blatantly tied to money rather than patient need?

An even bigger question is whether the scheme even worked. In fact, the numbers of people being diagnosed with dementia had already been rising well before the dementia-screening contract was introduced in 2013. There was no particular rise seen the following year,[48] meaning that although more people might have been getting referred to memory clinics there was no 'catch up' of diagnosing more people with dementia than might have been expected anyway. There were two other problems. First, a study in the *Lancet*, published after the screening was underway, showed that the true amount of dementia sufferers in the community was less than thought. In other words, fewer people were *'missing'* a diagnosis than had been been assumed.[49] Second, memory clinics became overwhelmed with new referrals, a consequence of false positive screening tests. Some neurologists wrote, dismayed by what was happening: *'... the incentivisation of diagnosis of dementia has the potential to make things worse.'*[50] People who really did have dementia would thus have waited longer to see a specialist at the memory clinic.

This incentives scheme was based on a political ideology, not evidence. Politicians rode it past the safety catches of the UK National Screening Committee. It was unpopular with patients and doctors, cost large sums of money and did not make a substantive increase in true dementia diagnosis – but probably did delay care for people who really did have dementia. It cost £42 million.[51] This was wasteful, damaging bad medicine, and for a bit of thought and humility could have been entirely avoided.

Financially incentivised medicine

The dementia-screening part of the contract is only a small part of an epic shift in how general practice works. GPs are paid through a patchwork of bit-part payments. A substantive part of GPs' money comes from Quality and Outcomes Payments – incentive payments on a massive scale. Every year these are renegotiated between the government and the British Medical Association and altered slightly (or, as a friend of mine put it: the contract hoops are moved higher and higher).

To start with, in 2003, the contract was reasonably straightforward. It rested on basic data gathering, such as keeping registers of how many patients had conditions like epilepsy or heart disease. The government had told the BMA, which had negotiated the contract, that it didn't expect GPs to score full contract points.[52] Instead, many GP practices got full or nearly full points and massive pay rises resulted,[53] with the average GP income up by 30%.

It was broadly accepted by the Department of Health and the medical trade unions that the pay of GPs until this point had been relatively too low, and part of the intention of the contract had been to raise earnings. But such a massive jump was unexpected.[54] Some analyses suggested that the Quality and Outcomes Framework (QOF) was a success, with more patients receiving recommended treatments, or better monitoring of their conditions. The second year of the contract was even better.[55] On the surface, it looked like GPs were being paid more to do more. Success?

Better recording of information was certainly achieved. Up till then, a doctor might have advised a patient to stop smoking but not bothered to write that down. Medical notes from 30 years ago usually show absolute brevity of note-taking. Often only the prescription is recorded, or just a diagnosis written, with no other information given. The contract began with financial rewards for filling in tick boxes. Smoker or not? Advice given to stop smoking or not? My memory of the first flush of the contract was of annoyance, like a mosquito in the room. I could get on with work more or less as normal, but had to remember to tick the boxes to prove what I had done.

The contract has since become more complex, more time consuming – and pedantic. For example, a glitch in the way the contract payments work means that entering data to code people as non-smokers or not has to be redone at regular intervals – even if someone has not taken up smoking in their 60 years. If a person was coded as having asthma between the ages of four and nine, and hasn't used an inhaler for a decade, the practice will be docked quality points if the person – who no longer has active asthma – does not have an annual check. To avoid this, doctors, practice managers and nurses have to continually review case files to ensure that the current codings are accurate. For this non-asthmatic person it would mean putting a new code in to say *diagnosis inactive*' or *asthma resolved*'. It does not affect the care a patient gets, only the income of the practice. Meantime, for people attending appointments to review conditions like bronchitis or heart disease, the use of large computer templates means that appointments have left many consultations resembling *'bureaucratic encounters, primarily oriented to completing data fields'.*[56]

Accurate records are a good idea – no question. Better coding benefits patients through research.[57] Collecting accurate data should allow better planning locally about how to staff specialist clinics and provide community resources. Practices can be compared and funding can be directed at areas of greater need.

However, the new emphasis on computer coding came with a cost. A research video analysis of GP consultations in 2004, when the contract was just getting going, concluded that the doctor's relationship with the computer often took priority over the relationship with the patient: *'... as tasks become more complex, they may become increasingly intrusive to the doctor–patient relationship, and in some cases may lead to a clinician apparently ignoring the patient and what they are saying.'* [58]

By 2010, the conflict between patient need and computer prompt was overbearing: *'Delaying entering some data until after the patient has left the consultation is an option, but the volume of data required for Quality and Outcomes Framework points means that we will almost certainly have to record some data while the patient is physically with us.'*[59] Separating patient needs from computer 'needs' had become practically impossible.

Another author has described the use of a computer in a personal interaction: *'Often it is as if the conversation has gained an additional participant, with whom only the user of the technology can communicate. The face-to-face conversation goes into suspense.'* [60] In the Netherlands, where there are many similarities with computer use in British GP surgeries, a two-phase video study was done, comparing consultations for high blood pressure in 1986 with consultations in 2002. In 1986 none of the doctors had a computer on their desk, whereas in 2002 all of them did. Doctors gave more medical information in 2002, but patients talked less and asked fewer questions. The main difference was new silences in the consultation, with the doctors spending an average of two minutes per patient entering computer data. In a ten-minute appointment, that's a substantive chunk of time.[61] The doctors were less likely to express concern about their patient and patients were less likely to express what was bothering them. And when we consider that almost one-third of patients left the GP surgery with unanswered questions about their condition, we should consider: who is being best served here? Another US study found that patients whose doctors used the computer more were less satisfied with their care, noting that the computer seemed to limit *'authentic engagement'.*[62]

The issue is that of opportunity cost, as described in Chapter 4. More data is being recorded. More boxes are being ticked. More points are being scored. But at what cost? What are we losing to make room for this? Can we have both – better recording and better quality of care?

In the UK, it was realised that the initial improvements that QOF seemed to deliver, before it evened out, were associated with a detrimental care in the conditions that did not have financial incentives attached to them.[63] Doing one thing with no extra resources meant less priority for something else – the slice of NHS cake was being redistributed. This may be okay if the priorities are correct – but are they? One doctor said, of the impact of QOF on the consultation: *'And there have been one or two occasions where I went through the cholesterol, the depression, the CHD (coronary heart disease), and everything else, and "Oh, that's wonderful, I'm finished now," and the patient said "Well, what about my foot then?" "What foot?"*[64] The patient gets the boxes ticked perfectly, but what the person actually wanted dealt with seems to have been pushed to last.

In the US, many hospitals have doctors whose pay rides on what procedures their patients have. Caesarian sections are more profitable than vaginal births. However, in general, in low-risk women, vaginal births are better for mother and baby.[65] What impact does this financial conflict of interest have? To answer this, a group of researchers examined doctors who were treating doctor-patients in hospitals in California during their own childbirth. They were able to compare hospitals with financial incentives for Caesarian sections to those with no such incentives. Hospitals with incentives had higher Caesarian rates overall. Doctor-patients, though, had fewer on average, with better outcomes for mother and baby. It seemed that doctors – who were likely to have had a high level of knowledge about risk and benefit of Caesarians – made different decisions about childbirth compared to others in the same hospital where there were financial incentives. They also had better outcomes.[66] Insider knowledge may trump the natural push of financial incentives – but what if you don't have that knowledge?

The apparent eclipse of QOF

The pressures of such unintended consequences and outcry from general practice became such that, in 2013, Jeremy Hunt proposed scrapping most QOF targets, saying: *'The 2004 GP contract broke the personal link between GP and patient. It piled target after target on doctors.'* He said that one-third of them would be removed.[67] GPs welcomed the news about changes to the contract, although there were new conditions and, effectively, pay cuts for older doctors. In Scotland, Shona Robinson, the health minister, told a conference of GPs, to thunderous applause, that she wanted QOF removed.[68] As I write, QOF has not gone in England.[69] While I hope it will eventually disappear, what is the evidence that incentive payments have worked at all?

The contract was introduced without a control group, and so it's impossible to compare what would naturally have happened without it. For example, there were incentive payments for encouraging adults to stop smoking and for increasing vaccination rates. Smoking rates did fall, but this happened in a wider context – laws on smoking in public places were also introduced, and smoking was already in decline.[70] The payment may have had some impact but it is very unlikely to have been the sole contributor. When it comes to vaccination schedules, there is pretty good evidence that incentive payments improve documentation.[71] Some anti-MMR vaccination websites have cited the payments made to GPs as a reason not to trust the recommendation (which is based on sound science) that children should be vaccinated. Would there have been more trust without the conflict of cash?

GP care was far from perfect when the contract was introduced. Some practices were badly organised, without efficient ways of managing people with long-term illnesses. Others were in buildings that were barely suitable, practices were badly staffed and postgraduate education was often erratic in delivery. More money into the service and better organisation is very likely to have made some positive difference to patients. But as the contract went beyond basic organisation into requiring numerous specific targets for blood pressure or diabetic control, it attempted to change a relationship between patient and doctor into a sequence of nano-management, orchestrated from Whitehall.

General practice, as we have seen, has had an uneasy relationship with its political masters. GPs did not become employees of the NHS when consultants did. Instead they have been contracted to the NHS to provide specified services. The resulting advantages have been a workforce free to organise locally as they saw fit, absorbing staffing and management pressures, taking responsibility in the main for the upkeep of their premises and rarely taking sick leave themselves. These were (and are) also the disadvantages. When, in 1950, the Collings Report stated that *'the overall state of general practice is bad and still deteriorating,'*[72] it led to a renaissance of sorts in general practice as many doctors took up the challenge to improve it. But this did not lead to GPs being brought into direct employment with the NHS. Over time, payments were made for specific, new *'items of service'* – for example, flu vaccinations and the number of women having cervical smears. By 1990, these items were explicitly called *'incentive targets'* with practices paid more once they had met higher thresholds.[73] In the *'new contract'* of 2004, the QOF meant the incentives had bred and grown wings.

What did the 2004 contract achieve? Did patients get better care and was it worth the sacrifices made, especially the impact of computers and increasing bureaucracy? This question is hard to answer. There have been no randomised controlled trials (though it would have been entirely possible to run them) showing the impact of the QOF contract. Instead, researchers have tracked what has happened to populations after the contract was introduced and used this to infer impact – it's a *yellow socks* situation. We should be cautious, therefore, about ascribing cause and effect, not simply because the contract hasn't been the only change that has occurred with the potential to affect the health of the nation, but because drugs started now, as a consequence of the contract, may only have a cumulative impact in five or ten years time. There is some evidence that people with diseases that were part of the contract (such as chronic obstructive airways disease or heart failure) were less likely to be admitted to hospital after, compared with before, the contract was put in place.[74] The contract may have contributed to this, but so many other changes have occurred – for example, outreach heart-failure nurses, *'hospital at home'* community respiratory teams – that it isn't possible to ascribe it to the contract. Another study examined whether those practices scoring high QOF points were less likely to have premature deaths among their patients compared to lower-scoring ones, and no relationship was found over the five years of the study.[75] Additionally, there is evidence that clinical care for people with asthma or heart disease was improving before the contract was introduced.[76] And the contract came with costs – not least a disruption to continuity of care.

When Hunt declared in 2013 that the era of QOF as integral to practice funding was over, there was a rare moment of political and GP unity. But instead of it being an indication that incentive payments were no way to organise systems, they were retained and expanded. For example, in an attempt to reduce the rate of A&E attendances, practices were paid to *'case manage'* a proportion of patients at high risk of using emergency services. NHS England – as also happened in Scotland – decided that it wanted 2% of all patients to be case-managed.[77] Thinking ahead and making plans for what kind of care is and isn't wanted by a patient and their family is often a good idea. Knowing about allergies, previous problems with treatment or circumstances that may make a person unwell and less able to make good choices is valuable information. Make a plan into a target, though, and there is a shift in values: it is being done because it is of financial value to the doctor, not (primarily) because it is of value to the patient. Some patients may be asked to make an advance plan, which – to them – is of little or no value but is (financially) to the doctor, representing a misuse of both parties' resources. Nor is there good evidence that advance care planning will reduce emergency hospital care,[78] yet the scheme was designed to save money and stop *'avoidable emergency hospital admissions'*.[79] The planning forms were meant to highlight to patients what actions they could take themselves rather than going into hospital. But everything that doctors do with good intentions can also cause harm, and I was concerned that all I was doing was inducing guilt in people who knew that if they did have a flare-up of an illness they were going to need expensive hospital care.

Whether doctors work better when there is a financial incentive is an argument that dates back to the birth of the NHS. Remember those two doctors, Bourne and Hill, back in 1943? Dr Bourne argued for a *'regular salary'* as opposed to intermittent fees from private patients. Dr Hill disagreed, claiming that what was needed was better organisation: *'I see no reason whatever to bring doctors into the position of the civil service as full-time officers.'*[80] Martin Roland, GP and professor of health research who has examined modern-day financial incentives, concluded in a letter to the *BMJ*:

'Financial incentives work, but not usually as well as those who introduce them hope for. Financial incentives can also have perverse or unintended consequences. Both of these are clear from extensive published research … If you were a patient, would you really want to visit a GP thinking that his next skiing

holiday might depend on him not referring you to a specialist? If variation in GPs' rates of referral is a problem, there are better ways of dealing with it.' [81]

In 2014, an analysis of the impact of ten years of QOF found that improvements accelerated initially but then fell back to where they would have been expected to get to without it. The researchers could not be sure that it was cost-effective.[82] Another study, published in the *BMJ* in 2015, concluded that there was no relationship between GP practices achieving high points and reductions in premature mortality.[83] We cannot reliably find that incentives have given long-term benefits to patients. Of course, with a short-term political cycle only interested in a short-term improvement, this might not matter if you are keen simply on soundbites and quick happenings. If we want a sustainable NHS for the next 100 years – not throwing away money, time or effort and ensuring that harms are minimised – organising doctors activity for incentive payments, as a Cochrane review concluded, does not come with enough evidence to tell us whether it does good or harm.[84]

The message from researchers is of incentives causing uncertainty and harm – we cannot be reasonably sure that the push to incentivise GPs for individual items of care represents either good value for taxpayers or better care for patients. We already knew that there wasn't enough evidence to roll out incentive schemes when they were pushed on GPs; we already knew that dementia screening didn't work and did harm even as GPs were being given money to do so. This is an absurd way to manage patient care, money and staff time. What's worse still is that the pattern had been recognised as foolish by the then government's official political opposition. The Labour Party was in power in 2008, when the Conservative Party stated: *'Their bureaucratic approach, running our health service through perpetual political interference and the imposition of top-down targets, is failing patients and undermining hard-working doctors and nurses. Originally introduced to provide accountability within the system, Labour's bureaucratic regime has created a situation where sticking to arbitrary targets (which often focus on*

*predetermined processes with little medical benefit) has become
more important than improving the health of patients. This target-
driven approach diverts precious time and money from genuine
clinical priorities. ... There is a wealth of evidence that targets
distort clinical priorities, lead to worse outcomes for patients
and have produced a demoralised workforce whose expertise in
delivering healthcare is constantly second-guessed.'* [85]

Yet that is exactly what has continued to happen.

The four-hour target

In 2004, the Labour government created a four-hour target
for treatment in A&E. It was under extreme pressure,
underfunded and long corridor waits were common. Money
was poured in to upgrade departments, train and hire more
staff, and change the way departments worked in order to
make the entire process faster. The original target was for
100% of patients to be admitted, transferred or discharged
after four hours – changed to 98% after negotiation. The
investment was welcomed, but in one survey 82% of A&E
doctors thought that clinical care had been adversely affected
– for example, moving people out before they were ready to do
so, or someone needing attention because they were about to
'*breach*' the four-hour wait, meaning that perhaps care was not
going faster to someone in greater medical need.[86]

Of course, it would be nice if everyone could get seen by
a professional within moments of opening the doors of A&E,
and discharged without having to resort to a magazine in a
waiting room. But the principle is of needs before wants. It is
entirely correct that someone with life-threatening injuries – a
heart attack, stroke or meningitis – should get seen quickly
and before someone else attending, say, for a second opinion
about chronic knee pain, or because someone has broken a
beauty nail accessory, or because they didn't want to wait a
few days to see their GP about a non-urgent problem.[87] Just as
Bevan talked about making the weekly budget last for seven
days: we all have to use the NHS wisely. The four-hour target
committed a cardinal sin in breaching that understanding: a

sustainable NHS should mean that the community agrees to prioritise each other according to need, not convenience.

What about imposed targets causing harm? In 2006, it was reported that hospital managers faced the sack if they failed to achieve the targets. However, *'gaming'* of the system was rife – for example, parking an ambulance outside the hospital (when the clock hadn't yet started), or even deliberately delaying ambulances to meet other targets set for ambulance response times, until the patient was no longer in danger of breaching the four-hour target.[88] But all we have done is repeat the same kinds of policy, somehow expecting different results. In 2016 the same problem was still occurring – 20,000 patients in south England were found to have had their ambulance to hospital deliberately delayed in order to help the hospital reach targets for ambulances. Yet a ten minute delay is critical.[89]

In 2008, the four-hour target for people to be discharged or moved out of the A&E departments came in for particular criticism in the Conservative Green Paper. Chapter 2 has already shown how targets in the mid-2000s made the care that people got in Mid Staffordshire worse, as well as making work more stressful and distressing for staff. The Green Paper – as cited earlier – stated that the Conservatives wanted to get rid of targets in the NHS, allowing professionals to be responsive to patient needs with the intention that: *'Any reason to structure activity around the interests of politicians simply falls away.'*[90] It was pointed out that the four-hour target: *'... is often cited for creating major distortions of clinical priority [and] ... has led to reduced average waiting times in A&E, but at the expense of patient care.'* It was correct that the policy was leading to the admission of patients unnecessarily as well as patients in high need of medical care being moved into less appropriate beds, yet the Conservative health secretary, Jeremy Hunt, was in the habit of phoning the chief executives of those hospitals that were not meeting the four-hour targets.[91] (It is worth remembering that the average length of service of a hospital chief executive in the UK is 30 months, as compared to the decades commonly served stateside: with pressures like these, it's not hard to see why.[92])

Big data, ratings and *'choices'*

A major component of the coalition government's (2010–2015) health strategy was patient choice. In 2011, the conservative party health secretary, Andrew Lansley, wrote that *'we will end the bureaucracy and top-down dictates of politically inspired targets'* and will *'provide information to support greater patient control over their healthcare and to facilitate choice of hospital and healthcare provider'.*[93] Choice has to be a good thing, surely? How could the opposite – force – be palatable, never mind appropriate? Being able to choose your doctor or hospital seems simply humane; why should someone be packed off to a medic who is patronising, uncaring or you just don't like? Why shouldn't you have a choice?

Any potential downsides of what might happen with *'choice'* went mainly unsaid. Instead, the political imperative was about how this should be got on and done. This would be through information, bucketloads of information.

The policy went on: *'Choice is made real through empowering patients, and patients are empowered if they have the right information. Patients know this; they want to access information but it is often not provided. Almost two-thirds of patients are unaware before they visit a GP that they have a choice of hospitals for first appointment. More specifically, patients should be able to obtain information not just about the choice of providers but about their condition, what to expect, what will happen to them, who will treat them, who they can ask about their care, and how they can have a say, or control, over their care.'*

To achieve this, Lansley described a new NHS Information Strategy, which would create *'a real market-place in information intermediation'.* He wanted potential patients to have information on standardised mortality rates – the death rates of patients surgeons had operated on, but with the numbers adjusted up or down to take account of how old or sick their patients were; and morbidity data, for example the number of blood clots after surgery, patient satisfaction survey scores and outcomes on surgery as reported by patients.

Releasing more information was not simply about enabling more patient choice – it was also a *'driver for clinical excellence'*,[94] as Lansley told a gathering of cardiothoracic surgeons. The Royal College of Surgeons agreed, saying: *'Patients are being denied access to real choice in treatment because the medical profession and NHS are dragging their feet on providing reliable, independent and accessible information.'*[95]

For the NHS to collect and analyse information about its own services is not, as a concept, new. For years, groups of enthusiastic NHS staff have shared data with each other to work out what they were doing or to compare services in different areas. For example, in 1995 the Renal Registry started gathering computerised data about kidney patients, and it aimed to share knowledge and plan future need for services.[96] In 1987, the clinical research practice Datalink started gathering information from GP practice records about illness, medicine and death rates.[97] What was different about Lansley's ideas was twofold: first, to generate data for the purposes of reselling it; and second, to use this data for new purposes. Rather than the data being a starting point to understand what the NHS was doing, the data was to be used to judge the quality of NHS services. Lansley's idea was that patients could use data about complication and death rates to choose the best surgeon. By the time it was published under the coalition government, the data was more clearly being used to force sections of the NHS to compete with each other. And, when the CQC was formed in 2009, the datasets gathered as part of the GP contract and used by the CQC to effect judgement, were used to compare practices and grade them into *'outstanding'* at the top and *'failed'* at the bottom.

Who could argue against transparency? Why should doctors have access to information about services while denying that to patients, perpetuating inequality in their relationship? And if a GP practice is doing badly compared to its peers, it would be unethical to stop patients from knowing that, so that they might decide to move from that practice to a better one.

Principles are important in medicine, just as they are in life. The idea of doctors collecting information about patients, services or their own performance but then locking it up and keeping it secret is abhorrent: being transparent about what medicine is doing and what happens when we do it is a fundamentally correct moral act. We should be able to tell whether one GP surgery has double the death rate of another surgery nearby; or whether one surgeon in particular does an out-of-date operation compared to his or her peers.

It is, though, a leap to suppose that this data will, as the coalition put it, result in: '... *ensuring greater transparency in the NHS and enabling patients to make informed choices about their care ... Patients will be free to choose the consultant team best placed to meet their individual needs and deliver the best possible results for them. Patients might choose a named consultant-led team which has the most experience of a particular condition or treatment on the advice of their GP, while others may choose to be treated by the consultant who has treated them successfully in the past.'* [98]

Where is the evidence? How do we know that the vision of data driving better care works, first, to improve services, and, second, to help patients get better care? The history of medicine is like a disaster movie with recurrent sequels. Bloodletting killed and maimed because testing the theory did not occur to the doctors who were enthusiastic about it and trained in providing it. Diethylstilbestrol has harmed generations of women and their children – entirely needlessly, for had randomised controlled trials been carried out before it was prescribed to millions of women the harms would have been spotted and the drug blacklisted sooner. When Vioxx was promoted by a $100 million annual marketing campaign in the US,[99] sales reps were told not to respond to doctors' questions about safety.[100] Urging patients to make a choice of surgeons based on data could be good; it could be bad; it could have mixed results. It may be popular; it may be unpopular; it may have unintended consequences. The principle of pushing out more accessible data became conflated with making choices on the basis of the data. The principle – transparency – was sound, but the policy – using data as touchstones by which to make choices about treatments – was unproven.

A trial would be the sensible thing to do. Take two health boards, for example, and leave one alone as a comparison group. Promote the use of surgeons' data for patients who are going to have surgery. Find out whether patients' access to this resulted in better operations, more confidence, improved recovery times and so on, or whether it resulted in more anxious patients, more worried doctors or surgeons who stopped taking on high-risk patients for fear it would make their numbers look bad. It took Samer Nashef, the author of *The Naked Surgeon*, to question his colleagues in cardiothoracic surgery and ask them whether any had stopped taking on high-risk patients because of concerns about their placing in league tables.

He told Radio 4: '*It has had an impact on surgeons. Surgeons are human, and if their results are going to be in the public domain, then consciously or unconsciously they will try to do something to make their results look good. I have surveyed the surgeons in the UK and asked them a couple of questions regarding this. For example, a question about whether they perhaps avoid operating on high-risk patients, with an eye over their shoulder to their figures. When I asked them that, about 30% said yes, they have done that, even though they knew that an operation was in the best interest of the patient, and perhaps more alarmingly, when I asked them whether they were aware of other surgeons doing this, the figure went up to 82% ... So there are downsides to transparency. And we have to say that the results of heart surgery in the UK overall are excellent and compare extremely well with the best international standards.*' [101]

It is bizarre that a new policy of lining up data designed to be used for comparisons was launched without any way to even tabulate the harms, never mind assess whether those harms were worthwhile accruing for the benefits.

In 2016, years after the data started to be published, academics along with the charity Sense about Science set about creating better information for readers of the data, explaining that if a hospital's survival rate is below its predicted range, it need not indicate alarm, but rather serves as a trigger for further investigation:

'There are four possible reasons why a hospital might be outside its predicted range:
- inaccurate or incomplete data
- the formula used to calculate the predicted range doesn't work well for that specific hospital
- chance (1 time in 20). (However, if you look at all 13 hospitals that carry out children's heart surgery at once, at least one hospital will fall outside its range just by chance about 9 times in 20.)
- because the chances of survival at that hospital are different to what is predicted.'

Despite this, a hospital had been temporarily closed due to faulty reading of earlier data.

Jeremy Hunt said: 'But my views are clear, and I set them out when I first got this job – my obligation is to follow the scientific evidence and spend the NHS's money on what is proven to work.' When he uttered those words was he then able to put aside his political lens when interpreting scientific evidence?[103]

It would appear not. There is a major problem. The practice of medicine has accepted the need to search for evidence and harms of interventions rather than relying on the prestige of job titles or egos as a reliable way to care for patients. Yet the NHS can still be forced into non-evidence-based, harmful interventions because policy can be dropped in without a set of brakes. We are not safeguarded by it being routinely tested and trialled, yet harmful policy can do just as much harm as bad medicine.

Allyson Pollock
professor of public health research and policy

I was working in Newham Health Authority as a senior registrar in public health, in 1988, looking at routine sources of data, when I suddenly realised that the NHS-provided community care services, including day centres for older and learning-disabled people, were shrinking. Social care, rehabilitation, support for older people in the community was disappearing. But the needs were not.

This started alarm bells going. When the 1990 'Working for Patients' White Paper was published it really affirmed my concerns. It was the start of the internal market and I had no doubts that it would ruin the comprehensive nature of NHS care we had. We had been studying economics, market competition, and market competition and choice, and Kenneth Arrow's seminal texts written 50 years earlier on why healthcare could not be delivered through the market.

I then started to look in more depth, with others, at the funding and provision of NHS and local authority services for people with long-term needs. Local authority-provided care was closing and being replaced by privately operated, for-profit, residential and nursing care homes. Long-stay bed provision was also closing and hospitals sold off. Under the rubric of care in the community, care was being transferred from the NHS to local authorities. This was a shift in care from being free at the point of delivery to NHS means-tested care, and a shift from public provision to private provision. The boundaries between health and social care had always been fudged; however, the 1990 NHS and Community Care Act shifted the boundaries between health and social care so that, increasingly, long-term care was means-tested and a local authority, not NHS, responsibility. This created huge discontent and a feeling of betrayal for people who had been promised 'cradle-to-grave' care. The Labour government did not implement the key recommendations of the majority report of the Royal Commission on long-term care.

Until the 90s, there had been no NHS 'providers' – just NHS 'services'. But with Thatcher's internal market, we had a different language – pricing, competition, choice, the creation of Trusts, and each with their own balance sheets. These hospitals and services were now stand alone corporate bodies having to compete for patients and money against each other. Then in 2012 we had the Health and Social Care Act (HSCA). Before this, the Secretary of State for Health had a duty to provide health services throughout England. That duty was abolished by the HSCA. Clinical commissioning groups (CCGs) locally have a duty to arrange services for the persons for whom they are responsible – but there is no duty to provide services for all residents in their area now. This creates a huge problem for local accountability and democracy. In future, it is possible that areas of the country and residents will have limited access to A&E or GP, or hospital services. Providers will decide for themselves where best to locate or run services or what it is profitable to provide – not necessarily what is needed and where.

Markets always try to limit their risks. In the US healthcare market, insurers and providers select out poor people, elderly people, homeless people, migrants, folk with mental illness and cherry pick the ones that they want. When I worked in the US the insurance companies' strategies for avoiding risk were well documented – like making older people walk up several flights of stairs before deciding who should get insurances. Running health services by private companies makes it about protecting shareholders, and selecting people out for risk and ability to pay.

Markets also bring huge new transactions. They bring costs the public sector doesn't have. We have never needed to advertise the NHS. In the US, healthcare providers spend a great deal of their budget on marketing their service and health plans – in the US, administration, communications contracts, billing, commercial contracts and so on can take up to 40% of the total budget. The public sector doesn't have to do any of that.

Where is this all going?

There would be a public outcry if the government had moved wholesale to privatisation. So, instead, we have another case of blurred boundaries. The market infrastructure and bureaucracy is *established for more and more privatisation – in fact, the HSCA requires all Trusts to become Foundation Trusts and allows Foundation Trusts to earn 49% of their income from private work. Hundreds of contracts – an increasing number – have gone to the private sector.*

Foundation Trusts and Trusts are in deficit – there is £20 billion to be saved from the NHS. So how are they to balance their books? Commissioning groups can reduce the volume of services they contract for and Monitor expects Foundation Trusts to reduce the NHS services they provide. Combined with the fact that NHS Foundation Trusts have been allowed increased capacity for doing more private work may mean that only the privately insured can get healthcare. This is extraordinary.

Many private contracts are for community-based services, services that deal with the most vulnerable people – prisoners, people with mental illness and learning disabilities. It ends up now that someone with a serious mental illness may have to travel hundreds of miles to receive care. These are a direct consequence of cuts and closures and the ideology of competition instead of needs-based provision.

It's a public health disaster. It shouldn't be like this. All the evidence shows that it is not possible to deliver universal healthcare through a market system. That is why the NHS, premised on public ownership and public funding, has been seen as among the fairest most efficient healthcare systems in the world.

When I first qualified as a junior doctor I had a sense of wonder when I walked onto my ward and looked after my patients. There was the wife of a judge in the next bed to a lollipop lady. The NHS is a great social leveller. That sense of wonderment has never left me. Having spent a year in America I have seen at first hand the effect of the constant fear of healthcare bills, and a lack of health insurance influences all sorts of decisions. When I went to see my own GP last week I queued alongside everyone else in the waiting room. The surgery is fantastic; it is located in one of the most deprived places in London; it is an oasis. Here I was – middle class and privileged – but I knew that the asylum seeker and poor immigrants sitting opposite me would receive the same care and attention and free at the point of delivery. That was what Bevan always intended.

6

Wrecking *'Reforms'* to the NHS

In the original *Star Wars* (1977) there is a planet-sized weapon known as the Death Star. In *Star Wars: The Force Awakens* (2016), a weapon 100 times bigger dwarfs the Death Star into puny miniature. The Health and Social Care Act of 2012 was much the same thing. The little Death Star of Lansley's competition and choice was replaced by a colossus.

The legislation in 2012 known as the Health and Social Care Act (HSCA) clashes fundamentally with the principles the service was built on. It made the government responsible for commissioning care, not for delivering it. GPs were no longer able to do the job they trained for – medical practice – but were to decide and commission the services to buy for their patients. Wales and Northern Ireland are not governed by the HSCA, and neither is Scotland, with the NHS now devolved to the Scottish parliament.[1]

The HSCA meant that commissioned services should be opened up to competition from *'any qualified provider'* in or out of the NHS. It meant GPs were changing role: instead of trying – at least in theory – to sort out the best way to organise services for patients locally, they were compelled to become arbiters, judging those organisations tendering and competing to supply services and award contracts.[2] This opened the NHS to a fragmented marketplace disarray of bit-piece players and profit-seeking enterprises[3] – exactly the messy, broken-up service problem that the NHS was set up to get away from. As a direct consequence of the HSCA, organisations like Capita, Circle and Virgin tendered and won contracts to run NHS services. These same companies have also terminated their contracts early, risking destabilising patient services as they did so.

Nicolas Timmins has described the HSCA – *'arguably the biggest structural upheaval in the health service's history'* – as *'a "car crash" of both politics and policy making'.*[4] NICE would have less ability to nationally recommend what was cost-effective and what was not, leaving individual commissioners to decide. There was no appeal to either academic evidence or historical memory to ensure that mistakes were not being created or repeated unnecessarily. The Health and Social Care Bill was contested by the BMA, the Keep Our NHS Public campaign, several Royal Colleges and numerous well-known and high-profile doctors and political campaigners. Richard Horton, editor of the *Lancet*, wrote *'We are about to see a phase of unprecedented chaos in our health services.'*[5] The editors of *Nursing Times*, the *Health Service Journal* and the *BMJ* wrote a joint editorial criticising it.[6] The government wrote a risk register of potential harms, but the final version was never published.[7] Leaks included a suggestion that the HSCA may push costs up through more private sector provision.

Opposition to the Bill even came from within the Conservative Party, with Norman Tebbit writing: *'In my time I have seen many efforts to create competition between state-owned airlines, car factories and steel makers. They all came unstuck. The unfairnesses were not all one way and they spring from the fact that state-owned and financed businesses and private sector ones are different animals.'* Not only do private hospitals not have to do any teaching or training, he explained, but the NHS hospitals *'cannot refuse to treat patients. Whether it is a drunken fool with a cut face from a street brawl, or a young mother with cancer or a heart attack, no one can be turned away, but the private hospital can pick and choose.'*[8] If fines were placed on the NHS, for example, for failing to give patients single-sex wards (as had been done) those fines would have to be met from somewhere within existing budgets and would inevitably impact on patient care.

Despite the protests, and a *'pause'* – supposedly for

a *'listening exercise'* [9] – the Bill received royal assent in March 2012. The HSCA duly created a *'brave new world'* of commissioning and competition, overseen by a new organisation called Monitor, and – as with the world envisaged by Aldous Huxley – it is a dystopia. The philosophy behind the HSCA embraced the concept of patient choice, in the belief that this would drive up standards. The invisible hand of free markets, it was believed, would improve quality and decrease costs – a development (or advancement) of the internal market of GP fundholding. Yet this is a philosophy, not a proven concept, and it makes a mockery of an evidence-based NHS. We should want a relationship between patients and healthcare professionals that is transparent and honest, yet the market-led process of commissioning, competition and tendering is rife with secretively cosy scandals of risk-free profit and conflicts of interest. As I write, there are increasing disparities in what local areas will pay for, with patients being increasingly disabled by conditions like cataracts before being allowed NHS surgery[10] as budgets are squeezed by cuts. Patients, when asked in research studies, cherish long-term relationships with their healthcare professionals, whereas competition encourages a systematic, short-term hurly-burly as contracts are won or lost. Rather than decisions being made with the use of evidence, an appreciation of uncertainty, a realisation of history and acknowledgement of the potential for harm, academic experts have been eschewed for the lure of expensive management consultancies. Glossy brochures from management consultancies have been used to persuade policymakers that efficiency savings can be easily and widely made. But instead of saving money, outsourcing in the era of the HSCA has driven costs up. The NHS has become more indebted, despite record historic expenditure and budgets.

The backstory

In 2005 a book called *Direct Democracy: An Agenda for a New Model Party* was published. The book's authors included Jeremy Hunt, Douglas Carswell, Michael Gove and Chris

Heaton-Harris.

'In five years' time Britain will have one of the most expensive health services in the world, second only to the USA', it was claimed. The authors argued: *'...the great challenge of our times is the need to reform those institutions which exist to serve the public interest in a way which makes them truly responsive to public demands and better fitted to advance the highest ideals of the liberal democratic West.'* In fact, UK spending on health as a percentage of GDP has been below the European average since before 1997[11] and below countries like the US, Sweden, Portugal, Canada and Denmark.[12] But the NHS constitution pivots on *'free at the point of need',* it does not revolve around *'public demands'.*

As David Cameron had done, these politicians bemoaned the fact that doctors had to *'chase meaningless targets set by the NHS quangos that run the health service, whilst patients wait months for operations'.* That is, of course, exactly what their government did. Their premise was that despite the money being spent, the NHS would be: *'... one which still fails to meet public expectations. The problem with the NHS is not one of resources. Rather, it is that the system remains a centrally run, state monopoly, designed over half a century ago... We should fund patients, either through the tax system or by way of universal insurance, to purchase healthcare from the provider of their choice. Those without means would have their contributions supplemented or paid for by the state.'*

They would do this via a government which was *'no longer a monopoly producer but instead acts as the funder and regulator'* using *'patient power'* to drive competition for *'speed, quality and choice'.* This competition would *'drive up standards',* using the latest technology and drugs.[13] No wonder, then, that in 2015 Hunt refused to guarantee that charges for some NHS services would not be introduced[14] – a recurrently mooted idea[15] that has floated around right-wing think tanks for years. This would fit entirely with their stated aim to *'break down the barriers between private and public provision, in effect denationalising the provision of health care in Britain'.*

And so in 2016, Hunt said, in response to the rationing of cataract operations *'Any patient who needs cataract treatment should get it without delay. Decisions about who gets treatment should always be clinically-led, and patients can pursue their right to ask for an alternative provider if they haven't started treatment within 18 weeks of referral.'* [16] This would appear to be crystallisation of ambition, for *'alternative providers'* will be found outwith the NHS.

The HSCA resulted in GPs having to set up clinical commissioning groups to buy in services from others. These groups would control an incredible two-thirds of the NHS budget while at the same time being given duties in quality improvement in general practice.[17] Would this benefit patients, ensure the NHS kept to its founding values or be cost-effective? To understand the likely repercussions we need to go back to the earlier attempt to make GPs responsible for buying in services, GP Fundholding.

Commissioning and competition in the internal market

In 1989, the White Paper *Working for Patients* was published, heralding the creation of the internal market through the National Health Service and Community Care Act of 1990. The NHS had previously decided what services it needed and supplied them. After the 1990 Act, it could buy those services in. Ken Clarke then introduced the 'purchaser/provider split', which took effect in 1991.

GP Fundholding was an opt-in scheme which around half of GPs took up before it was abolished in 1999. GPs were given a budget to buy services for their patients, and were mainly allowed to keep the remainder for improvements in their own practice. It was introduced without being piloted, evaluated or evidenced, and even several years after it started, there was no evidence about whether it has improved or worsened the quality of care.[18] According to Nigel Lawson, then Chancellor, it was the *'first step towards creating a genuine internal market within the Health Service'*. He has written that the lack of trials was an advantage because only people who were enthusiastic and chose to do so would get involved. However, this creates a performance bias, and is likely to skew the results.[19] Just as Trusts had to prove they were capable of becoming *'Foundation Trusts'*, GPs who wanted to be fundholders had to supply business management plans and show that they were good managers before being allowed to fundhold.[20] Research published just before the scheme was disbanded concluded: *'The major deficiency concerns any effect on health outcomes that may be the result of fundholding. Until such research is conducted, the jury will have to remain out on whether fundholding has secured improved efficiency in the delivery of health care.'* [21] Although researchers found evidence that waiting lists could be shortened by fundholding, many fundholding doctors complained that they could not improve clinical care for their patients.[22] Worryingly, patients of fundholding practices appeared less satisfied with their care and the costs of managing the processes needed were substantial.[23] As Iona Heath, previous president of the Royal College of GPs, has said: *'... we had a partner at the time, and I remember him arguing, and saying "it either advantages my patients at the expense of other doctors' patients, in which case it's immoral, or it doesn't in which case it's not worth the effort".'* [24] Despite almost a decade, millions of pounds and lives at stake, there was no prospective scientific attempt from the politicians to answer clearly whether this vast reorganisation into fundholding improved healthcare or made it worse.[25] Instead, answers were sought retrospectively, well after the policy was made and the money spent. The fundholding experiment was pure politics and no structure was in place to find out whether it did more harm than benefit for us. How could this be good for our society?

The responsibility for commissioning in the NHS was rolled back into Primary Care Trusts in the late 1990s, but in 2005 *'practice-based'* commissioning began.[26] The same mistakes looked likely. *'Policymakers do not seem to have learned the lessons from fundholding,'* wrote two academics.[27]

Practice-based commissioning had several commonalities with fundholding and did not resolve the core problem, which was identified in an article in the *BMJ* in 2005: '... *the commissioning general practitioner (or nurse) has to deal with a perennial tension: on the one hand being the agent for the individual patient and on the other being the guardian of resources for a wider population of patients.*' [28] As Heath identifies, this is a conflict with the underlying values of the NHS, which is for everyone. Instead of untangling the conflicts, however, commissioning compounded them. GPs are certainly used to dealing with one patient at a time, while being mindful of the resources they have to call on in the community: that's why generic prescriptions are used in preference to more expensive branded ones, and why referrals to hospital are prioritised to ensure the people in need of most urgent care go first. Commissioning a set of resources for a larger group of patients is beyond this, and often more about rationing than it is about clinical care. (And rationing is exactly what happened, as I will describe.)

Although practice-based commissioning was described as popular, take up was slow; it was competing for attention with other targets the managers had been set, such as the maximum 18-week wait for hospital appointments.[29] Financial incentives were even used in some areas to encourage it, allowing GPs to improve their own premises or equipment. But there was still a lack of evidence around whether better quality resulted – and since smaller, busier practices in poorer areas tended to be less involved in commissioning,[30] it meant that if there were advantages from it, then there was the possibility that wider health inequalities would result. A team from Bristol University explored the quality of care by searching for data on the effects of competition on the survival rates from heart attacks, and it revealed that in the early nineties: '*We find the impact of competition is to reduce quality. Hospitals located in more competitive areas have higher death rates during the period.*'[31] And in any case, even if competition was beneficial, people having heart attacks are unlikely to be in a position to make a thorough assessment of their choices of location for treatment; instead, the priority would be to take them quickly to the nearest necessarily equipped hospital. If, as the study found, more competition was detrimental, this is more likely to be due to systemic factors – such as where funds were being spent.

Cost but no benefits – the ISTC scandal

In parallel, competition was being used more widely and openly in hospital services. In 2003, the Labour government launched Independent Sector Treatment Centres (ISTCs). The centres used the private sector to do batches of operations (or, in phase 2 of the scheme, diagnostic scans such as CT or MRI scans). The ISTC scheme cost almost £5 billion, used multiple private providers and was deeply controversial. There was evidence that the centres were effectively *cherry picking* patients who needed more straightforward care,[32] meaning that they were being paid the same per procedure as the NHS, despite the NHS's patients being more complex and needing more care and attention. Phase 1 was run on *take or pay* contracts, meaning that even if the service was not used the NHS still had to pay for it – and the payment that had to be made to centres was above the standard NHS cost. The actual numbers were not revealed, on the grounds of *commercial confidentiality*,[33] even to the House of Commons Health Select Committee on request.[34] Taxpayers' money was thus poured in, even if the NHS got nothing back in return. Six private companies were given nearly £60 million in compensation for cancelled NHS contracts.[35] While one study claimed that ISTC were as good or even slightly better, it was not a fair comparison.[36]

One surgeon remarked upon the fact that it was a highly protected environment compared to the NHS: *'In an ISTC the surgeon and anaesthetist cannot be distracted by needs of patients other than those on their operating list – in stark contrast to what happens in the traditional NHS model. Surgeons in ISTCs are unlikely to find their operating list disrupted to treat an emergency that needs urgent surgery. The attention of surgeons and anaesthetists in ISTCs is not distracted by them having to teach medical students and mentor junior medical staff. And on the wards of these ISTCs the nursing staff are focused only on the needs of those having some very specific surgery – no need to be distracted by patients with complex medical and social conditions.'* [37]

In other words, comparing ISTCs with the NHS was not really about comparing apples and pears, but a fire extinguisher with a fire engine. ISTCs, given their resources, should have been far better than the NHS, but they were not.

GPs were also concerned about standards of care in some units. In 2005 both orthopaedic surgeons and ophthalmologists raised concerns about the lack of safety data. In one region there was a need for repeat surgery in 18% of its patients compared to under 1% in the NHS[38] – a problem not only for patients but also the NHS, which had to meet the cost of fixing the problems that resulted. Training for surgeons was cut back as a result of the ISTCs, because there were no junior doctors gaining experience under the tutelage of consultants in the private sector.[39] In short, the private sector profited and the NHS bore the consequences. Bear in mind that ISTCs were meant to increase capacity and choice: *'introduce best practice and innovation'* and *'through the challenge of competition from ISTCs, stimulate reform and improve efficiency in the NHS'.*[40]

The House of Commons Health Select Committee could find no evidence that any of this had happened. Indeed, in 2010 it commented that: *'... a number of witnesses argued that we have had the disadvantages of an adversarial system without as yet seeing many benefits from the purchaser/provider split. If reliable figures for the costs of commissioning prove that it is uneconomic and if it does not begin to improve soon, after 20 years of costly failure, the purchaser/provider split may need to be abolished.'* [41]

One can almost hear the scraping of deckchairs being shuffled around the Titanic. At what point does one have to say: this isn't working? Proving a negative is impossible – I can't prove that a chorus of singing goldfish won't appear on my desk tomorrow. But I can say that there is theoretical and practical evidence that reforms based on competition aren't working, along with the observation that since it hasn't happened yet in the 70-plus years of the NHS, it is very unlikely to.

Where is this all going? The publication of the *'Five Year Forward View in England'*[42] in 2016 promised more funding for general practice in order to alleviate *'unprecedented pressure'*. While the resources were welcome, £45 million was earmarked to *'stimulate online consultations systems'*, despite the lack of evidence this would be safer or save money or time. People with *'minor ailments'* are to be directed to online resources, and GPs are to do more online as people with non-medical qualifications take over some GP work.[43] Evidence was absent. It also directed GPs to work *'at scale'* in bigger practice set-ups, integrating social care and health care – already happening in Scotland.[44] This would seem entirely sensible – it is impossible to cleave apart social from health care needs – and has been done in limited ways before, but without clear evaluations.[45] Indeed, the evidence for cost effectiveness and harms seems weak or absent.[46]

Evidence-based medicine, as we have seen in the earlier chapters, should work by gathering all current data and then assessing it in an unbiased manner. Science starts at the null hypothesis. We assume our intervention does not work, and then look, in as careful a way as possible, for any signs that it does, and what harms it also creates. This is how to get progress: stop things that don't work, keep the things that do, look out for harms and, based on that, make fully informed choices as to whether they are worth it.

The health marketplace

Hold on: what did we already know about the effects of competition on healthcare? Was the HSCA based on evidence? After all, healthcare in the US, ruled by the market, is the most expensive system in the world – and one of the least cost-effective.[47]

In the words of Consumer Reports: *'... if our $3 trillion*

health care sector were its own country, it would be the world's fifth-largest economy.' US healthcare costs are double – double – the typical costs in other developed countries.[48] In 2013, 17.1% of the US GDP got spent on healthcare – 50% more than the next most expensive, France,[49] and it was 17.5% in 2014.[50]

What does the US get for its money? More. More scans, more tests, more interventions – 2.5 times more MRI scans, three times as many mammograms and one-third more caesarian sections.[51] A day in hospital in the US costs over ten times as much as in other countries.[52] This is absurd, and is bad, bad medicine; more is not better, it is worse. It represents overtreatment and side effects from needless treatments. Medicine is driven by profit-making practices rather than by doctors sharing risk and uncertainty with patients; regulation happens through litigation, meaning that the risk for the doctor is displaced to the patient, who is, through overinvestigation and treatment, bequeathed a financial and medical burden. The bottom line is that the US has a lower life expectancy compared to other OECD countries,[53] despite its comparatively lower tobacco and alcohol use. The US has a ferociously complex healthcare market, ruled by insurance companies, co-payments, competing hospitals and thundering advertising. The word I hear most when talking to US doctors, physicians and economists about their healthcare is *'chaos'.* The second most common word is *'waste'.*

Marketplaces do indeed work for many types of produce. Value for money can be tested in the part of the population willing to buy, with more expensive (better-quality or improved) items offered to those who can afford them, and cheaper (though possibly inferior) products offered to folk lower down the ladder. Advertising can be used to lure people into buying things they don't necessarily want or need. The manufacturers don't lie, but they don't have motivation to be honest – for example, about engine emissions, the likelihood of benefit in the real world, or the fact that a competitor has a better product. Products will only be made if they have a chance of selling and therefore be profitable, which means that niche items are unlikely to make the grade. If those are made, they will be extra expensive. The healthcare market has similar characteristics. People who have complicated or uncommon needs are less well catered for because they are less profitable. People can be sold interventions on the basis of misleading advertising that does not explain marginal benefits or harms fairly. More resources go to the people who are easiest to care for – rather than being allocated to people with the greatest needs. Market places are not reliable arbiters of distributive justice.

Markets for healthcare are deeply problematic. Take the case of Joclyn Krevat, a 32-year-old occupational therapist from New York City who was up to date with her health insurance. She suddenly became very ill, requiring an emergency heart transplant. She had it done at a hospital in her health plan's network of hospitals, but the transplant surgeons working there did not accept her insurance. She ended up with a bill for $70,000, and when still convalescing the debt collectors arrived.[54] She had not checked the small print of her insurance policy when she was critically unwell. Is this compassionate? Caring? The sort of society we would like to become? Are these the kinds of side effects from marketing healthcare that we are prepared to accept? Repeated studies have shown that US medical debt is borne not just by the poorest in society but mainly by middle-class people living in nice houses; a significant proportion of the public's debt – somewhere between half[55] and a quarter[56] – is associated with medical bills or illness. This is the fallout of an insurance-based system. It costs. Another consequence of the free market in the US is that there are financial incentives for doctors to do *more medicine*, which has led to high costs and low value, as people get tests and investigations they don't need while hospitals and doctors profit. In response to this, the Choosing Wisely campaign[57] has tried to inform patients about the risks and costs of overtreatment and pleaded for a way to *wind back the harms of too much medicine*.

Former registrar at St Thomas' Hospital in London, British politician and life peer David Owen, has also pointed out the flaws of believing in a *'market'* in health: *'The patient–doctor and patient–nurse relationships are personal, intimate and largely unquantifiable. The moment the patient believes that the decisions of doctors and nurses are being taken on cost grounds as the result of competitive trading the relationship of trust will alter ... Health is not a market commodity.'* [58]

This is not a new discovery. We have known about the problems of markets in healthcare for decades. In 1963, the US economist and Nobel Prize winner Kenneth Arrow – interviewed earlier (see pages 85–88) – wrote candidly in *Uncertainty and the Welfare Economics of Medical Care*, his seminal article on the economics of the healthcare market: *'That risk and uncertainty are, in fact, significant elements in medical care hardly needs argument. I will hold that virtually all the special features of this industry, in fact, stem from the prevalence of uncertainty.'* Such *'special features'* placed healthcare in a different bracket from other commodities. The demand for medical services due to illness is individually unpredictable, and as an *'assault on personal integrity'*, he wrote, it is *'a costly risk in itself'*. Doctors should act not out of popularity, but out of an ethical duty to do the right thing, not the easy or popular thing. Doctors should divorce their self-interest from patient interest – *'it is socially expected that this concern for the correct conveying of information will, when appropriate outweigh his desire to please his customer'*. In concluding, he writes: *'... the failure of the market to insure against uncertainties has created many social institutions in which the usual assumptions of the market are to some extent contradicted.'* In other words, the market system is not a good model for supplying healthcare because of the very things that make markets work: upping supply (for example, health screening that is not based in evidence and may only harm customers); advertising (because claims can be overstated or *'gamed'*); or cost (because recommendations are made based on clinical need, not ability to pay).[59]

Although Arrow has been criticised by some contemporary economists, who believe the answer is even more marketisation rather than less,[60] the death rates in the US or the cost of healthcare compared to other similar nations are unarguable. Other economists have suggested the opposite: that competition on price could make outcomes – death rates – worse,[61] especially when quality is not as transparent.

The NHS Confederation, which represents a wide range of organisations within the NHS, including commissioners, has written: *'Economic theory predicts that price competition is likely to lead to declining quality where (as in healthcare) quality is harder to observe than price. Evidence from price competition in the 1990s internal market and in cost-constrained markets in the US confirms this, with falling prices and reduced quality, particularly in harder-to-observe measures.'* [62]

(It is notable that, as Arrow says in his interview on pages 85–88, buying healthcare is not like buying fruit. Yet Roy Griffiths[63] and, later, Stuart Rose[64] were commissioned to advise the NHS – managers with backgrounds in Sainsbury's and Marks and Spencer, respectively.)

Although it would be very difficult, it would not be impossible to test the theories of those economists via randomised controlled trials. In any case, within the UK, we have an uncontrolled and unrandomised trial of what happens by comparing England with what happens in the other UK nations not under the jurisdiction of the HSCA. It's clear that economic or political theory is simply that; evidence of theories put into practice is what one should really want, and yet a succession of health ministers did not even suggest trialling their ideas. Nigel Lawson wrote in his autobiography about setting up the internal market in the NHS: *'There was much criticism when the White Paper was published that the Government was being characteristically doctrinaire and arrogant in imposing its reforms without even having a series of pilot projects. I found this very puzzling.'* [65] Similarly, Andrew Lansley has said of the HSCA: *'At the end of the day you have to say, "Did it work?" The long run – in so far as it was designed to create long-running stability for the NHS in terms of structures and powers – we will only know in 10 years' time.'* [66] In neither reflection is there any sense of needing to gather evidence, reflect on harms, or consider real-life problems before the rollout of unproven policy.

When the Conservative–Liberal Democrat coalition came to office in 2010 it published a White Paper, *Liberating the NHS*, the harbinger of the Health and Social Care Act, which promised to free the NHS from inefficient micromanagement of meeting targets and associated performance-management bureaucracy.[67] It declared its intention to abolish the then structure of commissioning through Primary Care Trusts and entrust groups of GPs with commissioning instead. Rather than winding back the healthcare market, the new government proposed to ramp it up. What was the evidence that such a proposal would deliver better clinical care or the improved cost-effectiveness that was desired? In 2012, academics from the University of York examined similar schemes for evidence of whether GPs would be effective commissioners and concluded: *'There is little evidence to suggest that GPs will succeed where others have failed and a risk that, without top-down performance management, service improvement will be patchy, leading to greater, not reduced, inequity.'* [68]

Not only the thesis – that markets would lead to better healthcare – was lacking in evidence, but so was the practical means of having GPs commission it. Furthermore, conflicts of interest created in these scenarios are rife: in 2015 it was found that 20% of GPs on commissioning groups had a financial stake in a provider they could commission to do the work – and this was not their own practice, but another, separate, provider.[69] The White Paper was not a systematic review of current knowledge. It did not analyse the harms, the uncertainties and the unknowns. Instead, political philosophy, not tested practice, was being used to overhaul the massively complex, enormous NHS organism. The underlying principle of the NHS was being changed – the buck no longer stopped with the secretary of state. The theory was that choice would drive competition, and competition would drive quality. But it did not examine the evidence.

Competition, choice and ratings

Within the HSCA environment, it soon became apparent that the tendering rounds for commissioning would have to be done within the bounds of European anti-competition law. The new chair of Monitor, David Bennett, told the *Times*: *'We, in the UK, have done this in other sectors before. We did it in gas, we did it in power, we did it in telecoms … We've done it in rail, we've done it in water, so there's actually 20 years of experience in taking monopolistic, monolithic markets and providers and exposing them to economic regulation.'* [70]

The NHS was the equivalent *'monopoly supplier'*, not a point lost on him: *'How can you compare buying electricity with buying healthcare services? Of course they are different. I would say … there are important similarities and that's what convinces me that choice and competition will work in the NHS as they did in those other sectors.'* Monitor, the organisation now meant to oversee competition in the NHS *'would have concurrent powers (with the Office of Fair Trading) to apply competition law'*,[71] meaning that it could enforce anti-competitive behaviour between Trusts. Lawyers were advising Trusts that they needed to *'protect themselves against any suggestion that they are acting anti-competitively, and consider that competition-based complaints are unlikely to come from patients, but from other NHS services or providers who feel aggrieved or disadvantaged'*.[72] Bennett also told the FT that commissioners could *'think about rewriting contracts, about performance managing providers against their contracts more effectively, about providing more integrated care and about the possibility of a competitive process to secure the best possible provider'*.[73] How much of the NHS budget was now going to be spent on legal fees?

The means to drive this competitive market was patient choice, promoted by the coalition government as the *'right thing'* to do.[74] Through a complex system of hospitals and

GP surgeries being rated online and by the Care Quality Commission, the belief was that the public disclosure of ratings would direct patients towards successful institutions and away from the bad ones. The bad would have to up their game to survive, the good would have to get even better.[75] Initial proposals included the idea of having GP practices marked green, amber and red in accordance with how often elderly people were admitted to hospital (seen as a bad thing) or how often cancer was diagnosed (a high number was seen as a good thing).[76] Win, win.

Except: what is the evidence? How does this work in practice? What are the benefits? What are the harms? Choices about healthcare are often made for reasonable, practical purposes: to be near a relative to help with recovery or to avoid a side effect in order to have a higher quality of life. There is nothing new about this. It is normal, good medicine. Choosing clinics, surgeons or GPs on the basis of online ratings are something separate. It is most accessible to those who are technologically capable and who are not so unwell that they cannot shop around for the best 'deal'. People without these abilities – or advocacy on their behalf – have, in essence, to 'take what they get'. Some individuals may have too many other competing interests, or personal demands, in life to make searching and acting on this information a priority. Natural social justice would mean that we should protect the people with the least resources first, and concentrate efforts to ensure that no matter where a patient attends the service is good enough to meet their needs and treat them well.

Ratings systems pervert this desired outcome. Does a GP practice in a leafy suburb have the same chances of good ratings from its patients as a practice in a deprived urban borough with high crime and unemployment rates? Maybe well-off patients will be less satisfied with reasonable care and poor patients grateful for very little or substandard care? Better-funded practices, or practices more able to give more time to patients, may get better ratings even though the source of their superiority is dictated by governmental funding policies and not the individual actions of staff (and it's clear that practices in more deprived areas get less funding[77]). Would a GP practice marked red be tempted to admit patients less – even when they needed to go into hospital – just to make the figures look good?

'*How good is your doctor's surgery? Check using this new online service.*' [78] In the late 1990s, large national postal surveys were sent to GP patients. These surveys were tied to a financial incentive for doctors to respond to them.[79] Healthcare systems have to listen and respond to patients' needs and views – who else are they there to serve?[80] Indeed, the website patientopinion.org.uk has, for over a decade, collected stories (good and bad) about the NHS and helped teams to improve or reflect on what has happened. The same postal surveys continue in various incarnations.[81]

Using them to promote competition, as rating sites do, is different. There are several privately owned and run enterprises which list all UK registered doctors and then offer scoring systems to give doctors a mark and make comments. I've seen dead doctors registered, doctors who work in one city being listed in another and doctors being contemporarily rated even though they were on maternity leave at the time. What evidence is there that online ratings are reliable enough to enable people to make better choices about healthcare professionals or services? One review concluded '*there is little published research on improvements resulting from feedback information of patient satisfaction surveys and most often these studies are contradictory in their findings*'.[82] A study from Europe noted some links between doctors' online ratings and supposed quality measures from their clinical work, as did an overview of associations between hospital quality of care markers and positive online reviews.[83] However, there are many unknowns.[84] The crucial questions are: Do these ratings systems help poorer services do better? Do they help people make better choices? It isn't fair to judge a hospital as worse if it serves people with more needs but has fewer resources. If a better-rated hospital then takes staff away from the poorer one, these harms then have to be absorbed by another group of patients.

But where are the harms? Since the harms haven't been examined or quantified scientifically, I can offer only anecdote, this from the US. A South Carolina woman headed to her local emergency room with toothache. The doctor gave her '*Dilaudid, a powerful intramuscular narcotic typically reserved for cancer-related pain. Why, his nurse queried, was he killing a flea with a sledgehammer? Afraid of malpractice? No, the doctor replied, my (online) scores last month were low*'. Here we have overtreatment – with all the attendant harms – justified as a means to a better online rating from a patient.[85]

Another study has found a relationship between fewer antibiotics being prescribed and lower patient satisfaction scores.[86] Set in the context of official concerns over too much antibiotic prescribing it's easy to see that doctors rated as popular may be doing the wrong thing. From my own work I know that it's usually far, far easier, faster and less taxing to give out antibiotics even when they are very likely to do more harm than good. It takes longer, requires more effort and risks confrontation to do better medicine. A GP colleague was asked to provide a sick note that she felt wasn't warranted. This was followed by a verbal altercation and a hostile online review. She was upset and shaken. This may or may not have affected her consulting style, or her ability to confront with such difficult issues in the future. The principle of freedom of speech is still justified despite harm – her patient had the right to say what he wanted (even if, due to confidentiality, she had no right of reply). But what about the problem of gaming the system, as in the South Carolina example? Or patients who got antibiotics – whether they needed them or not – being more satisfied? Who is getting good care then? In 2016 a research paper examined the effect of private provision of hip surgery in the NHS in Scotland between 1993 and 2013. More private provision has been associated with a decrease in NHS provision with older people and people in the most deprived areas missing out – in other words, markets in medicine favour the already favoured.[87]

Management consultancies and conflicts

Management consultancies had been intricately involved with both the drawing up of the HSCA and its aftermath. At least one management consultant was suggesting that the insurance-based model, so beloved of the US, was keenly anticipated in the UK. The head of KPMG, Mark Britnell, said in 2011: *'GPs will have to aggregate purchasing power and there will be a big opportunity for those companies that can facilitate this process ... In future, the NHS will be a state insurance provider, not a state deliverer.'* He added: *'The NHS will be shown no mercy and the best time to take advantage of this will be in the next couple of years.'*

Anti-lobbying campaigners Spinwatch found evidence of communications between NHS managers (who would be involved in commissioning) and management consultancy companies, facilitated by a group that was in turn chaired by a lobbyist for UnitedHealth Group.[88] It is clear that prior to the passage of the HSCA, management consultants McKinsey were actively discussing the takeover of NHS hospitals by *'international hospital provider groups'*, which would be looking for *'a free hand with staff management'* ... *'if £500 million revenue (is) on the table'*.[89] It gets more complicated because UnitedHealth Group – along with Capita, KPMG and PricewaterhouseCoopers (PwC) – is an *'approved'* NHS supplier,[90] meaning that it is able to take commissioned contracts for GP or hospital services.

In 2013 I read a report by PwC purporting to show that technology in the NHS could save money.[91] I found that the report itself had cost £75,000, yet it was fatally flawed, scattered not just with typos but also with false assertions about the quoted evidence – for example, confusing inpatient stays with outpatient attendances, extrapolating widely from the management of rare conditions and making entirely non-evidence-based statements suggesting that large quantities of patients could be safely managed at home rather than in hospital.[92]

Using management consultants rather than academics to research efficiency savings and NHS planning has always struck me as odd. Academics are trained to justify their conclusions, state uncertainties and to progress an argument with logic and references. Management consultancy reports, in general, do not. The much-quoted McKinsey's report of 2009 about how the NHS could achieve *world class* NHS productivity savings of 22% over five years was similarly silly. They said District Nurses were *under performing* if they did less than the median of home visits; but they did not examine why. For example, the nurses could have been dealing with patients needing palliative care, or attending meetings with GPs about vulnerable adults – there was no explanation as to why the variability existed. In any case, McKinsey recommended that GPs who saw fewer patients should have shorter appointment times in order not to be such *weak performers*, which is bizarre, given that longer appointments are much preferred by GPs and patients, especially if the person has complex needs, and such appointments are standard for minor surgery or contraceptive fitting. And they assumed that GPs who referred their patients more to hospitals (or, as they put it, the *worst* GPs) should decrease referrals to become average and save money – without investigating whether these were rational referrals (or, indeed, whether other, under-averagely referring GPs could be considered to be under-referring).[93] Reports like these are simple analyses of big data, which make judgements about what the data means without understanding the clinical contexts or the subtleties of illness. Big data should be the beginning of a story to unpick meaning rather than being the end itself. There is no doubt that overtreatment happens in the NHS – jeez, I've written a book about it – but the question of where valuable savings can be made safely, compassionately and usefully needs far better interrogation.

The tentacles of management consultancies had reached far

and deep: they were involved in both making the law and then profiting from it, sitting on both sides of the commissioning and the commissioned divide, being hired to advise GP commissioning groups on how to spend the money.[94] GPs in London alone spent £7 million on management consultants supposedly to teach GPs business skills in commissioning.[95] This would, in any other circumstances, be regarded very seriously as a conflict of interest, so why not here? Further, what is the evidence that training of this kind is good use of taxpayers' money? In any case, it is a lot of capital to recoup; what kind of vision would be imparted at these sessions to make these kinds of savings? And how, with falling NHS budgets, could this be done in a way that would benefit rather than harm patient care? This industry is parasitical on the NHS. Barts Health NHS Trust spent almost £1 million on one management consultant over ten months in 2014.[96] The bill for management consultants in the NHS doubled between 2010 and 2014 from £313 million to £640 million – how can we afford this?[97]

David Bennett, the head of Monitor, had previously worked for McKinsey,[98] which stood to make much capital out of the new post-HSCA NHS. He and other members of Monitor had been criticised for accepting trips to New York and for attending leisure events for themselves and their families paid for by McKinsey. Indeed, 40% of Monitor's costs in 2012/13 – some £7.8 million – went to management consultants.[99]

Another notable feature of the new era in UK healthcare is the blurred 'revolving door' [100] for health ministers who move from politics into management consultancies and senior positions in health think tanks. Andrew Lansley became an associate of a management consultancy in 2015.[101] Simon Stevens, CEO of NHS England, previously spent a decade working for UnitedHealth Group,[102] which has tendered for many NHS contracts under the HSCA.[103] Stephen Dorrell, previously chair of the House of Commons Health Select Committee, is a senior advisor to KPMG.[104] Alan Milburn, a former Labour health secretary who signed contracts expanding the role of the private sector in the NHS,[105] owns AM Strategy, which does media/consultancy work.[106] Milburn has also received payments from PepsiCo[107] and is the chair of the online doctors' rating company iWantGreatCare, chair of PricewaterhouseCoopers' Health Industry Oversight Board (which advises their private health clients)[108] and chairs Bridgepoint Capital's European Advisory Board.[109] Bridgepoint is a major shareholder in Care UK. Patricia Hewitt, another Labour health secretary, afterwards took up roles with Boots and Cinven, which owns private hospitals.[110] Lord Hutton, who was previously a Labour health minister, took up posts advising PricewaterhouseCoopers and joined the board of Circle in 2014.[111] Conservative Sir Malcolm Rifkind sits on the board of Alliance Medical.[112] This tangled, messy web is full of potential conflicts of interest, well-paid consultancies, interconnecting spheres of unwritten influence and overlapping interests. In the private sector, Freedom of Information (FOI) requests don't apply, and no one will know what goes on in unminuted, unrecorded meetings behind closed doors. Is this really how we want the future of our publicly funded NHS to be decided?

But, on top of everything else, where is the evidence that management consultants themselves – to use their own phrase – can *'think out of the box'*? Which of them have ever assessed the harms and hazards their profession creates? Why do they almost always find that privatisation is a better solution, and why do they never question the evidence for the philosophy that their profits rest on? But most of all, as I have mentioned previously, where are the opinions of real experts? In the UK we have a fine network of academics with expertise in sociology, management, medicine, nursing, statistics and risk. Repeatedly, they produce independent reports showing that particular political policies were generated with little or no evidence of benefit and that they overlooked harms. Yet academic reports are inevitably produced after, and not before, money, time and energy are wasted implementing poorly evidenced and researched policy.

The NHS - stealth privatised and exploited

Has the HSCA resulted in privatisation? Virgin, Specsavers and Care UK were among 105 companies granted 'any qualified provider' status in 2013.[113] A succession of FOI requests published in the BMJ in 2014 found that private companies had been given one-third of the contracts awarded by commissioners since April 2013.[114] In 2015, the Department of Health released figures showing that private health spending had been 2.8% in 2006/7, 4.9% in 2010/11 and 6.1% in 2013/14.[115] While these figures lack context and detail, they show a clear direction. Despite the evidence that more contracts have gone and were going to private providers, the health secretary told parliament in 2015 that 'privatisation is not happening'.[116] Choosing not to call this privatisation would seem to be more to do with semantics.

The HSCA is not an overnight transformation wrought by a single government – the public–private direction of travel within the NHS has been signalled for some time. In a 2011 essay by James Meek in the London Review of Books, a surgeon described the complex joint replacement he was about to do: 'The case we're doing this morning, we're going to make a loss of about £5,000. The private sector wouldn't do it. ... How do we deal with that? Some procedures the ebitda [earnings before interest, taxation, depreciation and amortisation] is about 8%. If you make an ebitda of 12% you're making a real profit. ... Last year we did about 1,400 hip replacements ... The worrying thing for us is we lost a million pounds doing that. What we worked out is that our length of stay [the time patients spend in hospital after an operation] was six days. If we can get it down to five days we break even and if it's four, we make a million pound profit.'[117]

Since 2004, in order to achieve Foundation Trust status hospitals have had to balance their books. The hospitals would receive a set national tariff for various procedures, which would be identified via codes. There are two problems with this: the tariffs do not account for differences between patients; and they reward short stays, which may sometimes be detrimental for individual patients, and a longer stay would clearly mean that some procedures were not worth doing – in financial terms. Indeed, as the surgeon told Meek: '... the most important issue is the finance. We get a lot of money from the cheap and cheerful procedures, we take a hit on others. The managers are cool with that, as long as we're getting a reputation as a centre of orthopaedic excellence'. That may be okay, but it depends on the books remaining balanced and the patients having an agreeable manager and surgeon. It means that the 'choice' offered to the patient effectively isn't real, since a non-NHS hospital would not offer the treatment. It means that patients have to depend on a moral contract with the NHS rather than on a market-based economy to give them the healthcare that is needed.

There is a longer history of competitive tendering damaging the quality of healthcare. In 2008, Primary Care Trusts were commissioning care for sexual health services, and that year the British Association for Sexual Health and HIV (BASHH) and the Independent Advisory Group on Sexual Health and HIV surveyed some of their members. Sexual health doctors tend to work either on the periphery of hospitals or in community clinics. They deal almost entirely in outpatients, rather than needing hospital beds, and work closely with psychologists, infectious disease experts, laboratory staff, and often police liaison officers.

BASHH reported: *'Various themes were repeatedly mentioned such as clinical governance concerns, viability of services, collapse of perfectly good services, poor staff morale, lack of transparency, fairness (and legality) of the process, conflicts of interest, lack of consultation, exclusion from discussions, adversarial atmosphere with commissioners, lack of impact assessment and a general concern for the future of the specialty, sexual health training and sexual health outcomes in general. I do not recall a single positive comment.'*

Directors and leaders of the sexual health services in areas where competitive tendering occurred were overwhelmingly unhappy with the process. *'Just when we seem to be doing well (for example, with fast access) services are having to divert time and resources to combat tendering,'* said one. *'We train and supervise sexual health professionals, we innovate, we do research. Will commercial organisations take on these roles too?'* said another. Others talked about a *'dumbing down'* of clinics; for example, cheaper contracts were being offered by consortia via the replacement of higher qualified staff, or fewer consultants in the service. Some said it was an *'expensive, divisive and ineffective way to improve the services'* or just an *'extremely destructive process for all parties'.*[118] There is a sense of frustration, but also instability. Working relationships across specialities were being tested in competition, rather than there being a collaborative relationship as usual. Instead of clinics working together for their patients, they were being placed into a contest for patients. The time taken for the tender process was time that was removed from other aspects of work: the busiest services may have been least able to express their case – and explaining a business case would have been a step in the dark for most clinicians. *'It has taken me 15 years of diplomacy, tenacity and sheer hard work to build up this service but tendering can destroy services very quickly',* wrote one head of service.

These shortcomings were made much worse by the HCSA. In February 2012, Circle became the first private company to take over the running of an NHS hospital: Hitchingbrooke in Cambridgeshire. Circle had a ten-year contract, but it withdrew just three years in, saying it was underfunded and that demand for A&E had risen.[119] Even the year before the contract fell apart Circle was saying: *'... clinical outcomes remain very strong. The hospital is a success story.'* [120] Jeremy Hunt was unrepentant, tweeting: *'This* [government] *makes no apology for seeking solutions for failing hospitals. We won't be deterred from tackling poor care and driving up standards.'* But Hunt had said previously that he would act according to the evidence – so where was the evidence that spending money on commissioning services would result in better value or care for patients? The House of Commons Health Select Committee had stated in 2013: *'Circle's bid was not properly risk assessed and ... Circle was encouraged to submit overly optimistic and unachievable savings projections. While some financial and demand risk has been transferred to Circle, the NHS can never transfer the operational risk of running a hospital, leaving the taxpayer exposed should the franchise fail.'* [121]

Additionally, the National Audit Committee pointed out that under the terms of the contract, Circle would be responsible for only some of its debt – the taxpayer would be *'left exposed'* to pick up the rest. Not only that, the chief executive was given a generous redundancy package and left to work in another NHS role. What went wrong? Neither the management team nor the Trust board were held to account, as *'accountabilities and responsibilities are fragmented and dispersed'*.[122]

The terms of the HSCA means tendering, which means that competition and failure will be inevitable consequences for at least one party involved in the process. It is pointless for a watchdog or inquiry to insist retrospectively that *'learning must happen'* from mistakes in tendering or commissioning, when the problem is systemic. Tendering results in uncertainty for staff, changes to contracts, disruption of patient care and often a new round of tendering, the costs of which will all be met by the NHS and taxpayers.

For example, in late 2014, an NHS consortium fought off tenders from Virgin and Care UK to co-ordinate and run community older people's care in Cambridgeshire and Peterborough.[123] Serco, Capita and Circle had all pulled out of the tender for the deal during the process.[124] One company that withdrew from the bidding process told the FT *'the customer wanted to pass a budget deficit to the private sector with no real way of making it good'*. A portion of the money in the deal was to be withheld unless certain targets were met, such as reducing hospital admissions. After eight months, the deal – which was for £1.2 billion and was meant to last at least five and possibly seven years – collapsed. The tendering process itself was reported as having cost £1 million; this process cannot be seen as anything but a wasteful one, and with an outcome that was surely predictable, given the cost savings that were to be made in order to win the contract[125] – indeed, Monitor apparently signed off on the consortium's bid despite reports of *'grave doubts'* and numerous unresolved issues about the contract.[126] The National Audit Office noted that the wasted cost to the NHS of the contract set up and bidder costs was £8.9 million.[127] If a service can be run more efficiently, and therefore profitably, should that surplus not go back into public service? Social care cuts, as we have seen, press the NHS: neither can be comfortably separated. Pressure on one forces pressure on the other. Marketisation expects that a portion of tenders will fail; as Arrow says, this is a normal part of markets. For people who are in the middle of treatments or enjoy good relationships with their doctors, this instability is hazardous. Healthcare is primarily a service; it does not exist to do things cheaply but to do them well. A cheap tender may win a contract but will prove to be unsustainable. Corners have to be cut to make the promised savings and deliver a profit to shareholders.

There are numerous examples of private-sector companies winning contracts only to fail to deliver on some significant measure. For example, in 2006, Serco won the contract to supply night and weekend GP services in Cornwall. Whistleblowers complained that there were gaps in the rota and that the data that judged performance targets had been changed *'where there was no evidence to justify the change'*. Serco did not have enough skilled people working to deliver the services,[128] so the contract was stopped 17 months early, in 2013 rather than the contracted 2015, and reverted to a GP-led consortium.[129] Private company Mitie won a £90 million contract in Cornwall to deliver cleaning and catering to hospitals; however, sick rate costs went up almost sixfold[130] and a senior clinician raised concerns that staff were not adhering to basic hygiene practices.[131]

There is more. In 2009, Serco went into partnership with Guy's and St Thomas' NHS Trust after securing the contract for laboratory services, the unseen but vital part of the NHS where blood and tissue tests are performed, reported and audited, and the results communicated and often explained back to clinicians. Serco was performing 22 million tests a year, making profits of several million pounds annually, when auditors found it was routinely overcharging the NHS. Clinicians had also raised concerns that cost-cutting was leading to errors, and staff who left were either replaced with less-well-qualified personnel or not at all.[132] One clinician wrote, in an internal email raising concerns about the service, that the company had an 'inherent inability ... to understand that you cannot cut corners and put cost saving above quality'.[133]

In 2015, in Stoke, a bid from Alliance Medical – of Rifkind's association – won the £80 million pound contract to supply PET scans to people (usually with cancer) in the area, despite costing £7 million more than the NHS bid. Yet the PET/CT scanner to be used was owned by the university hospital and had been paid for partly with bequests and public donations.[134]

Margaret Hodge, chair of the Public Accounts Committee tweeted in September 2014: 'No rational person would do business with a company that cheated so why does govt?? [government] Because they have let G4S; serco get too big to fail.' [135]

HSCA's effects on general practice

The effect of the HSCA on GPs was that instead of remaining primarily clinicians, they turned into commissioners – without, as we have seen, any real evidence that this would be safe for or beneficial to patients. It also created a new type of GP: the practice-running entrepreneur. 'The Practice' in Brighton is owned by two GPs[136] who have gradually taken on more and more practices. However, in 2016 the pair – now running services for 11,500 people – terminated their contract early, citing funding pressures.[137] This destabilisation is felt hard by patients who don't know what will happen;

but this is not like buying vegetables, for when a group of practices fails there isn't another supplier around the corner with spare carrots.

Just as with the hospital sector, many private companies are now supplying services to GPs. Virgin Healthcare, as well as hospital contracts, now has 230 contracts to supply GP practices and social care services in England worth £500 million. Sir Richard Branson has said, of Virgin Care, that *using our entrepreneurial skills, it is possible to improve healthcare in the UK, and yet, save the taxpayer quite a lot of money*.[138] (However, tax research experts have noted that Virgin Care is one of about ten private health providers that use tax havens as part of their corporate structure, so taxpayers may actually beg to differ.[139])

Is Branson's claim true? How would we know? Companies like Virgin are not subject to FOI requests, and the public accountability that the NHS must have – for example, board meetings in partly in public – do not apply.[140] It's notable that one GP says in praise of his Virgin employer: *I feel empowered to deliver good quality care without the burden of an open-ended time commitment.* (Jobs also come with a discount card for Virgin trains.) Meanwhile, patients complained of a succession of locum rather than permanent doctors and Virgin had been found to try and meet targets by asking family and friends of staff to do sexual infection tests.[142] Virgin has also stepped away from contracts after being appointed the *preferred bidder*, allegedly when realising that the money on offer was not enough – and passing it back to the public sector.[143] In 2014, Clinical Commissioning Groups decided to put locally enhanced services – such as contraception or reviews for people on long-term medication – out to tender, and companies like Boots and Bupa were enthusiastic, with a director of Lloyds Pharmacy saying it would offer *efficient and cost-effective alternatives*.[144]

As the academic John Lister has put it: *Far from being put in charge, or "liberated", it is clear that GPs are simply being used as a handy lever to force through changes – and take the blame for the negative consequences.'* [145]

Indeed, the vast majority of GPs in one survey said they did not have the skills to commission safely.[146] And, inevitably, the result of commissioning has been *'postcode lotteries'* – the amount or type of services commissioned by GPs varying from area to area. So, in some places, bariatric surgery for very obese people is more available compared to others.[147] The gloss put on the restrictions of IVF, or changing the thresholds of allowing joint surgery, has been that such procedures are of limited use.[148] And while this may or may not be true, it begets two problems. The first is that there may be some benefits to some people, and the judgement to use an intervention is usually about weighing uncertainties. Prioritising strict rules above an appreciation of uncertainty may result in worse care. The second problem is of equity. Why should people living short distances apart, both living under the auspices of a National Health Service, be separated by the services available to them?

The long-term relationship that GPs and nurses used to have with their individual patients and practice as a whole is dissolving. Certainly, some improvements may have been made through some commissioning but this need not have taken a monumental Act of parliament to turn the NHS on its head while simultaneously ordering huge cost savings. The post-HSCA environment is a mess, a wholescale rocking of the boat – and not so much rocking it as threatening to sink it.

For most patients, general practice has traditionally been their front door into the NHS. Until 2004, GPs were responsible for making sure that their patients had recourse to a GP 24/7. The new GP contract changed this entirely. GPs were no longer responsible for ensuring that their patients had access to primary healthcare in the evenings and weekends because this task became legally the responsibility of Primary Care Trusts (PCTs). What happened subsequently demonstrates starkly the pitfalls of pursuing profit in the context of the healthcare market.

Until 2004, most GPs did their own on call work. Often

they would share a rota with a nearby surgery, meaning they were on call at least one evening and night during the week and then again at the weekend. There was no day off the next day. Over time, there was a change in the type of problems people phoned about. Call outs were no longer for grave things such as heart attacks, strokes or serious disease. Instead, people wanted urgent advice about matters like head lice, the feeding patterns of babies or to discuss a sprained ankle – things that would have kept safely until the next working day during the 1960s and 1970s. By the 1990s, there were still calls about serious – or potentially serious – illness, but there was also an increase in calls about conditions which would have been managed, decades before, at home and without advice from anyone outwith the family. Certainly, for many doctors, this mixture felt unsafe. In dealing with so many calls it was becoming easier to miss the really sick people waiting down the line. The moral contract that doctors had meant that they would work evenings, nights and weekends as well as daytime because there was a need for them to do so. As the kinds of requests for urgent advice changed, the motivations for doctors perhaps also changed. They felt they were no longer servicing acute and urgent need or medical emergencies. I've spoken to many GPs in their 60s and 70s who describe a sense of frustration: trying to organise a good death at home for an elderly person while callers complained of the wait to get a prescription for paracetamol. GPs were stressed and exhausted, and their families often felt short changed.

GPs then led on reorganising evening and weekend care on a bigger scale. Instead of sharing on call rotas with the practice down the road, GPs across whole towns and cities joined together. Work would be more intense, but better protected and administered, with shorter shifts (6 p.m. till midnight, or midnight till 7 a.m., rather than 6 p.m. to 7 a.m.), and with additional staff like nurses and drivers and telephonists to share some of the workload. These centres were great fun to work in, often designed for the purpose. But in 2004, the offer was made to GPs to give up their on call commitment for an annual price that worked out at somewhere between £6,000 and £9,000 each.

There is now a general agreement that this was grossly undervalued, but many PCTs seemed to think they could provide as good or better service for less money. This was exemplified by the contracts for some of these large centres being placed out to tender. While some areas of England – and, of course, the devolved nations – continued to provide not-for-profit co-operatives of GPs to share the evening, night and weekend working, other areas had the services taken over by private providers. Serco entered into talks with other providers to relinquish one contract early,[149] and in 2015 it was transferred back to more or less where it started.[150] Of course, if a company wins a bid by being £1 million a year cheaper – as Serco was – running costs have to be cut.[151] That usually means staff numbers or how qualified they are. There is concern for safety when such cuts are made.

The same pattern can be seen in urgent and out of hours centres across England. In Hackney, London, Harmoni won the contract but was using large amounts of agency staff and lacked enough GP cover. Harmoni had received multiple complaints about delays in the service as well as poor reviews from the CQC. A local group of GPs offered to take the service over in 2012, but the local commissioning board, afraid of litigation under competition law, decided that the process had to be open to full public tender.[152] Eventually, in 2013, the GPs took over the service[153] with one saying, *of course it's just going back to what was a very successful set-up, running for almost 20 years'.*

Huge amounts of money have been wasted as bits of the NHS fought with each other for emergency and urgent care scraps from the table. But something really important has also been lost. Before 2004, GPs had a sense of responsibility for their patients. The overwhelming nature of the unchecked demands placed on the service rendered it impossible for GPs to deliver. Change was necessary, but that change has come in the form of outsourcing, which has replaced a moral contract with a for-profit one. However, the financial market did not make it work: as the frequent gaps in the rota have made clear, doctors do not want to work in a stressful, unpleasant, uncontrolled environment. However, as the doctors in Hackney and Cornwall have shown, many doctors still have a desire to fulfil that duty of providing cover at nights and weekends – but only under different terms of financial, workplace and moral contract.

The NHS 111 fiasco

A vast amount of money and time has also been spent organising and then reorganising the NHS telephone advice line system. In 2013, the new 'NHS 111' service replaced the older NHS Direct, which was mainly staffed by nurses, and was a phone line for medical advice – what Alan Maynard described as *'an effort to try and reduce the demand on GPs and in A&E'*. NHS Direct cost £123 million a year and was popular with *'mothers and parents with children'*.[154] NHS 111 employed proportionately fewer nurses – an inevitability, when the intention was to reduce the cost of dealing with a call from £24 to around £10. Most calls are taken by call advisors with little training (adverts instead asked for typing and telesales skills) who are given a couple of weeks training. The impact on A&E was rapid. Indeed, pilots of NHS 111 had shown that 29 more ambulances were called per 1,000 calls compared to NHS Direct.[155] It was calculated that there were 450,000 extra attendances at A&E over the following year, and the blame was laid with NHS 111 for being too cautious in its advice.[156] Caution in medicine is often warranted, but it becomes counter-productive when this ends up producing life-threatening delays to other people who are more ill and in need of faster attention.

Clinicians had said that NHS 111 was not fit for purpose before it was rolled out.[157] Some of the NHS 111 contracts went to NHS ambulance Trusts, and others to private companies like Care UK. NHS Direct also won some, but then it withdrew in 2013, saying that the cost of running a nurse-heavy service exceeded the price that was being paid.[158] Having a lower proportion of nurses might make the service cheaper to run, but it was never going to make the service safer or more able to make clinical judgements. Call advisors work to a rigid protocol series of questions and answers that are designed to be used by someone with little clinical experience. But if there is no experience, clinical judgement, as a skill, hasn't been developed. It's far easier to order an ambulance than to make a reasonable judgement about whether someone needs to be taken immediately to hospital. Call handlers looking for clinical advice often didn't get it due to there being too few doctors on the ground.[159]

When NHS Direct withdrew from its 111 contract, new contracts for each area with new providers had to be tendered – at a cost of half a million pounds in one area alone.[160] Any money 'saved' by having given the original contract to a cheaper provider was simply moved towards paying legal and commissioning fees – money that was not spent on clinical care.

The transfer into 111 was not just about a new service, but a different service. I was walking through Euston Station in London when I saw a poster encouraging people aged over 60 to call 111 because 'minor illnesses can get worse quickly'. Another poster asked 'feeling under the weather?' and encouraged people to call; another had the smiling face of a middle-aged woman: 'Started the week with a sore throat that just wouldn't go away. By the weekend, I'd also got a high temperature and nasty headache. Called 111, who arranged an out of hours GP appointment for me. Back to my old self in no time – can't wait to catch up with the girls.'

I'd love to know what wonderful cure the GP had administered. This common set of winter symptoms sounds like a flu-like illness, and if this person phoned me for advice, there is a good chance that they wouldn't need seeing in person at all. The scene was being set: if you are not feeling very well you should phone and expect to be seen urgently and made to feel better. Is this realistic? Much of my work as a

GP is about explaining the options we have to operate within the limitations before us. Flu-like illnesses are nasty, but they don't need antibiotics. Viral coughs are unpleasant but they last almost three weeks.[161] These campaigns were health marketisation in another form. People were being asked to consider calling 111, even if they hadn't thought it was really necessary. Demand was being created. It is likely that NHS 111 thought that this campaign might stop people from becoming more unwell later on, but there is and was no evidence that these sorts of campaigns can do that. Instead, expectations were elevated to the heavens and beyond. As an analysis of the 111 service has found: *'There is potential that this type of service increases overall demand for urgent care.'* [162]

Is the only way to make the NHS sustainable to manage demand to increase healthcare supply but at a lower quality? There are two options: either increase supply or decrease demand.

Continuity of care and twisting targets

I should apologise for mentioning continuity of care again, but it's essential. It cannot be avoided in any discussion of demand or sustainability. For the last decade, the narrative on the NHS has pushed for rapid access to healthcare. In many circumstances this is entirely correct. For a heart attack, a stroke, a diabetic coma or a protracted seizure, it doesn't really matter what qualified healthcare professional you see. You want and need urgent care. But for many other people, it's more complicated. Half of GP appointments are taken up by the 29% of the population who have long-term conditions; this group accounts for 64% of outpatient appointments and needs 70% of NHS and social care spending.[163]

The number of people with multiple long-term conditions is increasing, and starts at a younger age in areas of deprivation. A typical patient in general practice is not a fit, healthy young woman who simply needs a renewal of her contraceptive. Instead, it is an older person with high blood pressure, obesity, diabetes and the beginnings of chronic bronchitis, who is on nine different medications, finds it hard to get out of the house due to immobility, and is frequently anxious and low in mood.

This kind of complexity is what GPs are specialists in: it's easy to see how breathlessness could be caused by the bronchitis, the obesity, anxiety, or a mixture of all three. It's plain as well that this person may need frequent medical care, and that a new doctor being involved each time will have to rapidly take account of an extensive amount of new information. This means that much of the consultation time would be spent on old information and not what the person needs to deal with today.

A patient and a doctor who know each other have a different set of ideals. The doctor knows that Mrs Harris's daughter is back using drugs, and that Mrs Harris is once again looking after her granddaughter. Her doctor knows that Mrs Harris is willing to do anything that will prevent her from going into hospital, and although the control of her diabetes might be thought 'poor', she had episodes of low blood sugar the last time her medication was increased and, on balance, the risk of overtreatment is currently worse than undertreatment. Mrs Harris knows that her current breathlessness is probably because she is having more panic attacks, but she has sought advice from her GP because two years ago she had a severe chest infection and she is keen to ensure another will not develop. This is not a one-off consultation, but another chapter in the longer story of her life, which intertwines with multiple and interacting events off stage. Because her GP knows what is happening elsewhere in Mrs Harris's life, the two of them can work together to address what is important (excluding a significant chest infection) while prioritising her wish to be at home to look after her grandchild, mindful of the fact that her anxiety levels are high, and is there anything that could help?

Continuity of care does not just result in better consultations for patients,[164] with patients generally preferring them[165] (the difference between 'my doctor' and 'a doctor'), it saves money. It is associated with decreased hospital admissions.[166] However, the state of medicine means that continuity is disrupted by systems which have not paid sufficient respect to it.

The 2004 contract brought the aim of *'fast access'* to GPs[167] within 48 hours.[168] Crucially, it was to be with *'any'* general practitioner. As I have mentioned, this is fine for many emergencies, but it was a new and untested way of running general practice. With no additional doctors, surgeries simply cut the cloth to fit. There were no more appointments. So appointments that could be booked in advance were reduced, in order to make sure there were enough available 48 hours ahead. If you have a chronic disease and need to make an appointment in advance, this is useless: you would have less chance of being able to book your review appointment with the doctor of your choice. The system pulled apart the seam of continuity that was being naturally woven. It uploaded stress, because patients had to ring the surgery at opening time and at the other end staff prepared themselves for a surge of calls. GP surgeries were awarded *'quality points'* (in other words, money) for keeping to the target. If surgeries failed to hit the target, then they could hand over the responsibility (and the money) to the Primary Care Trust, which could commission walk-in centres to do the 48-hour access work instead.[169] Patients didn't like how the 48-hour target worked; doctors didn't like it; and politicians didn't seem to know the on-the-ground consequences of the policies they expostulated. Doctors who had to go to training sessions to show them how to reach the target talked of how it felt like a *'cheat'*.[170] Tony Blair, taken aback by a description of how difficult the target had made it to get an appointment, said it was *'absurd'*.[171]

Yes, it was *'absurd'*, but also predictable.

Access targets get in the way, and not just in general practice. In 2016, an ambulance Trust was found to have *'downgraded'* 111 calls for ambulances in order to meet performance targets – even when clinical staff advised that this was not safe – and it only stopped doing so when whistleblowers spoke out.[172] This is immoral, but it is an example of how targets can crowd out basic ethical principles. Worse still is when targets set for fast access fail to realise the resources already present in general practice. Not only did systems already exist, but doctors already had a moral duty to see people who were in urgent need, regardless of how overbooked their surgeries already were (and not in 48 hours either: if there was urgent need, they would be seen quicker). The political imperative was for a top-down 'solution', but it ignored the biggest resource the NHS has: the people who work in it, and the people who use it.

The outrageous economics of PFI

Now, sure, we have to balance the books: but where could the money be safely saved? From front line patient care – as per David Cameron's letter – or avoiding wasteful policies? Stephen Dorrell, then Tory MP and chair of the Health Committee was clear: *'There is no precedent for efficiency gains on this scale in the history of the NHS. Nor has any precedent yet been found of any healthcare system anywhere in the world doing anything similar.'*[173]

However, one of the most catastrophic wastes of money has been the Private Finance Initiative (PFI) scheme, which is effectively the public sector taking a loan from the private sector. The tragedy is that this politically driven endeavour was predictably wasteful. PFI started under John Major's Conservative government and was continued by Labour and then the Coalition government.

The warning signs – of both the long-term and short-term cost of servicing repayments – were identified early on. The first of the new era of NHS hospitals built with private money was Guys Phase 3 development in 1986. Charities and other public sector agencies were going to use the building and contributed towards it. They were meant to contribute 45% of the overall cost of £32 million. However, delays, the insolvency of contractors, an increase in VAT and changes to building regulations put the end cost at £152 million. The partners did not pay the increased share and the NHS was left to pay their money as well. Under the 1990 Health and Community Care Act, hospital Trusts had to pay the cost of their capital, and thus had to make a 6% profit on their income over expenditure to pay back to the government. Moving capital off the balance sheet became a way to balance the books: less capital meant less return would have to be paid back.[174]

By April 2011, there were 700 PFI contracts in England alone worth £50 billion. PFI funding was used to build new hospitals and primary care venues, then service them – for example, with catering and cleaning. PFI offers large immediate sums of money from private investors, but borrowing rates are generally 2.5–4% above the rates that local authorities would otherwise be able to obtain, and the loans tend to be of the nature of 20 years and above, some even to 60-year terms.[175]

Between 1997 and 2008, despite cheaper loans being available to the NHS during this time, 90% of funds for hospital building were through PFI.[176] Allyson Pollock and her colleagues, writing in 1999, predicted what would happen: *'The private finance initiative is an expensive financial option and has brought with it severe affordability problems at both local and national level ... Under the private finance initiative the NHS pays more for less; paradoxically, the "largest hospital building programme in the history of the NHS" is being funded by the largest acute hospital closure programme.'* [177]

In 2010, the National Audit Office noted that *'there is no evidence that including these services in a PFI contract is better or worse value for money than managing them separately'*[178] and *'investors and contractors will naturally seek to maximise their profit margins, and we have seen examples where this is at the expense of the Trust'*. In 2011, the Treasury reported: *'The substantial increase in private finance costs means that the PFI financing method is now extremely inefficient.'* [179]

In 2014, Northumbria NHS Trust was the first to negotiate out of its PFI deal because it was crippled with PFI debt. The hospital had cost £51 million in 2003, but, including maintenance, £250 million would have been repaid over 32 years. The Trust bought out the debt via a loan from their local council, thereby saving £3.5 million a year.[180] Elsewhere, hospitals were crippled with PFI debts – in Peterborough the budget deficit was £40 million against PFI annual repayment of 42 million.[181]

Barts Health NHS Trust in London cost £1.1 billion in construction costs, but Barts will end up paying back £7.1 billion. In 2015/16 they will pay £127 million. Barts has been criticised for unsafely low nurse numbers; in 2015, it ran a deficit of £90 million. It will be in debt until 2049.[182]

So, yes, make efficiency savings. But let's put this into perspective. Efficiency savings were being made – but these were protecting PFI paybacks at the expense of direct patient care. None of this was unforeseen. Pollock and colleagues were writing about it from 1999 onwards: there were plenty of missed opportunities for policymakers to pay attention.[183]

Impossible sums

The state of the NHS as we approach the end of 2016 is perilous. There is simply not enough money being put in. Trusts are being paid less for procedures they do – and there will be a shortfall in England's NHS of £22 billion by 2021.[184]

Hospitals have already made sweeping efficiency savings: after that, it is front line services that are cut. Funding deficits have resulted in A&Es and maternity units being closed or stripped of services.[185]

General practices have found themselves in recruitment crises, going bust and/or unable to recruit staff.[186] One clinical commissioning group had even discussed forbidding GPs from making non-urgent referrals in a bid to save money.[187] Even Scotland, which has been protected from the worst of non-evidence-based policymaking in the form of the Health and Social Care Act 2012, has still been subject to austerity politics and has run up NHS deficits.[188] Of course, the other set of savings that can be made in the NHS is doing policy differently. How much of the NHS budget is wasted on non-evidence-based policymaking, which either causes overt waste, or simply harms patients and takes staff away from providing front line services? The Health and Social Care Act, serial NHS IT disasters including care.data, healthchecks, dementia screening, commissioning, operations like knee washouts at arthroscopy for arthritis, the care connect phone line – these are failures of policy making. Without a system to ensure that non-evidence-based policies are not allowed, money given to the NHS is at risk of being squandered on short term political ideas, not hard facts about cost-effectiveness. Front line staff shortages and raw resources have been eroded to meet the costs of projects that didn't help patients.

Otherwise, what will happen is the full utilisation of the HSCA. GPs will leave overpressured and understaffed permanent jobs, freelancing their services for private providers. Hospitals will restrict their services so that only people with private insurance or who can pay will receive certain treatments – as we are currently seeing with cataract surgery or joint replacements.[189] That this surgery can be done in NHS hospitals but on a private basis – as per the HSCA – adds insult to injury. This is how privatisation is done – not through a catastrophic sudden shudder through the NHS, but through a thousand tiny shockwaves, each an instability of its own, and by the time the public realises what is happening to our most compassionate of human endeavours, the NHS will be irreparable.

Professor John Appleby
chief economist, King's Fund

What's the right amount of money to spend on the NHS? Well, it's whatever we want to spend! The question really is what we're prepared to give up to spend our limited resources on the NHS. At some point we'll want to stop spending on the NHS and spend more on education, or on disposable income. It's difficult to judge where that switch from healthcare to other spending might occur.

We can see what other countries do. We spend more than Mexico, but less than Germany. Remember, we are the fifth or sixth largest economy in the world. As a proportion of our wealth, UK health spending is comparatively low – just over 8% of GDP. We don't spend as much as many other countries we might like to compare ourselves to – France, Sweden, Denmark or Belgium – which spend around 10% to 11% of their GDP on healthcare. We probably wouldn't want to spend as much as the US, which devotes about $1 in six to health (a big chunk of which is not spent efficiently).

As NHS funding has been squeezed lately relative to what needs to be spent, I would judge that there is also increasing public support for boosting funding.

Spending on the NHS has risen historically – on average around 4% more than inflation every year since 1948. But now it is in the middle of a decade-long squeeze where funding will only rise by an average of just under 1% a year. And NHS spending will lag behind growth in our GDP. Over the next few years we will find ourselves slipping down the spending league compared to our European neighbours.

This funding squeeze coupled with growing demand for healthcare has come to a head this year, 2016. Over 90% of English acute hospitals are spending more than they are getting in income. Big, well-run hospitals like the Royal Free or

University College Hospital in London will overspend this year. Overall, NHS providers could end up with a £2 billion to £3 billion deficit this year – equivalent to seven to ten days' running costs for the entire NHS.

Over time the NHS has managed to improve productivity, making its budget go further and do more. For example, switching from expensive branded drugs to cheaper generic equivalents. And the length of time patients stay in hospital has been cut through better surgical techniques and anaesthetics – allowing more patients to be treated with fewer beds. But these developments take time.

Competition has been one policy introduced in the 1990s to try and incentivise hospitals to improve their efficiency and quality. There is some evidence it has done so, but no one knows how cost-effective this 25-year-long experiment has been. It could be argued that competition has not been effective enough to prevent NHS providers running up deficits recently as funding growth slowed.

But nor has competition led to the wholesale privatisation of the provision of NHS care some feared. Of course, the NHS is paid for by public money but buys in many things from the private market – drugs, buildings, architects. And a significant chunk of healthcare has always been privately provided under contract to the NHS – such as general practice. I don't have an ideological objection to private providers. The important point is whether the NHS is paid for in an equitable way, that patients have a universal right of access and that they are protected in times of service failure – which can happen both in the public and private sectors.

Ensuring high-quality services – whether publicly or privately provided – isn't easy. The original PFI contracts, for example, were generally not good value for the NHS. But the NHS learned to negotiate better deals latterly. Competition isn't a costless exercise; there are legal and administrative costs of contracting. Clinical commissioning groups can seem to be wasting money on tendering services. But such transaction costs (including the 'costs' of private providers' profits) need to be offset against the benefits of such a process. Unfortunately, as I have said, while there have been some estimates of costs and some evaluations of benefits, there has been no comprehensive evaluation of the policy of competition as a whole.

It is not just the NHS that is under pressure financially at the moment. Social care has taken a real battering over the last five or six years and looks set to suffer more in this parliament. A big chunk of social care provision is private and local authorities have tried to squeeze as much as they can from the deals they strike with private care home providers in the face of big real cuts to their budgets. But now the private market in nursing homes is teetering on the edge financially. The prices local authorities are offering to pay mean that many care homes are not sure they can deliver adequate services.

Local authorities have a statutory duty to provide care, but the squeeze on their budgets is enormous. Care staff have increasingly seen their pay shrink as providers try and meet the contract offers from local authorities. But the introduction of the national living wage – a good thing – adds to care home costs of course. The worry is that care homes will go out of business and local authorities won't be able to cope. A lack of social care places and higher thresholds for other social care services is shifting an increasingly large burden onto vulnerable and frail elderly people and their families. It also has knock-on effects for the NHS, with hospital discharges being delayed and – anecdotally at least – increased use of emergency services that could have been avoided with better social care arrangements.

7

Humans in a Digital NHS

In the NHS humans are cared for by other humans, who are as all humans are: flawed, prone to fatigue and capable of making mistakes even when well intentioned. This chapter examines how those workers are trained, trusted, organised, valued and managed; and how they are equipped to do their work to best effect. Human care is the obvious thing lacking when the NHS goes wrong – from careless staff to murderous Harold Shipman – but the systems that are meant to support health workers and the stresses upon them are often invisible. In truth, the waste of resources is both human and financial. The training of staff has moved from 'on-trust' to 'by-proof', but comes with no evidence that this recipe for doctor-making is any better. The NHS is hampered by astonishingly poor-value IT programmes and labyrinthine referral systems, which have been used to produce more big data of questionable value. The drive for more data as evidence of improved efficiency, proficiency, 'customer' satisfaction levels and cost-efficiency has produced a management culture of inspections and regulation which have become so burdensome that it has contributed, paradoxically, to the staff feeling devalued and untrusted. Humans with humane values are working in a healthcare system that often acknowledges neither.

The NHS is a human endeavour. We all make mistakes, but those in the NHS can cost lives as well as money and time. Mistakes harm patients, and often have profound effects on the staff who make them. Too few staff, and pressures on staff time are a risk factor for mistakes, yet there is scant attention given to safe staffing. Rather than organisational decisions being made on the best available evidence, new policies are routinely launched without considering the impact on the people who serve the NHS.

Training and trust

When I was a medical student, it was necessary to assist at ten births in order to *'pass'* the undergraduate Obstetrics and Gynaecology exam. We had cards that had to be signed to prove that we had attended the births claimed on our tick sheet. They were half-checked by our seniors, but it would have been simple to counterfeit, lie or *'lose'* the card, or otherwise get around the stipulation. It was *'trust-heavy'* and *'regulation-light'*.

As a junior, there were complaints that senior house officers (SHOs) – one step up from first year house doctors – were a *'the lost tribe'*.[1] The charge was that they could spend many years in SHO grade before finding a registrar post. One could try out multiple specialities and hospitals, accumulating experience and knowledge before completing registrar and senior registrar grades and becoming a consultant. These junior doctor posts were not brilliantly paid and would normally come with a heavy on call rota. There was a bottleneck to get into registrar grade posts. The Department of Health launched a programme called Modernising Medical Careers, which was to be centrally administered and intended to streamline careers. Despite advance warnings that the computer system wasn't capable of handling the applications, the Medical Training Application Service (MTAS) was launched in 2007, whereupon the computer systems repeatedly broke down. CVs had to be standardised, and points which were scored for various achievements were widely seen as unfair.[2] Further, personal details of some doctors were accidentally made public.[3] There were marches in protest. The 2008 Tooke Report into MTAS said not only was doctors' involvement in training policymaking *'weak'* but that: *'Policy development should be evidence led where such evidence exists and evidence must be sought where it does not.'* Amen to that! Further, the report found 'evidence of DH [Department of Health] deficiencies in policymaking with ambiguous accountability structures for policy development, and very weak governance and risk management processes'.[4]

There is no doubt that some junior doctors had been exploited for low pay and long hours, with little opportunity to progress in their careers. But the answer to that problem was not an excessively bureaucratic, distant and disorganised process that produced accidentally unemployed junior doctors, sweat, tears and disrupted careers. It was organising without evidence, thoughtful consideration or enough consultation with doctors themselves. An entire industry has bloomed around the regulation and revalidation of doctors, monitoring them and deciding whether they can return to practice in the UK. Even doctors who have trained in the UK and have worked in similar healthcare organisations abroad only for short periods of time are often subject to costly, time-consuming processes before they are allowed to return to work – ironic, given the shortages.

Appraisal and revalidation

When I started in practice, we were expected to go along to postgraduate meetings and generally keep ourselves up to date. Points were awarded per hour of education, and these were totted up over the year to show that the required threshold had been met.[5] There was enjoyment in attending meetings with fellow staff. This easy socialisation boosted morale and the cross-pollination of ideas and practice – like a giant coffee time. It was relatively easy to keep up with contemporary practice and to quiz our colleagues and experts. It was not burdensome. It was rather nice.

We now have annual appraisal, and every five years, if one has 'passed' each, you are allowed to revalidate – essentially, keeping your license to practice medicine. It didn't always look like this: a series of medical scandals focused regulators' minds and the 'solution' was appraisal. So now I am meant to write down everything that I look up or learn as 'proof' that

I am a good doctor. I have to spend evenings writing up my *'reflections'* on what I have learned and what I am planning to learn next, and then I have to explain myself if I do not achieve it.

And what are the harms? Firstly, time. On average, 12 to 15 hours are spent completing the paperwork and appraisal, the forms are unwieldy, and GPs, when asked, describe how the professional learning is valuable but the appraisal far less so.[6] Added up across the nation, this is a sizeable chunk of doctors' time being shifted from patient care into paperwork.

Secondly, there is the statutory collection of feedback. The General Medical Council (GMC) has a list of surveys which we have to ask our patients to complete and which they deem acceptable, and GPs have to pay for these, one way or another. Appraisal is now an expanded business empire, but where is the evidence that it is useful? A 360-degree feedback is the beloved buzzword. Many GPs now pay companies to gather and analyse feedback for them. The GMC requests 50 patient feedback sheets for revalidation.[7] Yet there is a dearth of evidence to show either the cost-effectiveness of this or that it leads to improvement beyond good working practices like regular breaks to talk work over with colleagues. (Or, as the educationalists would have it: active peer review and reflection.)

Appraisal has progressed into an extravaganza. I have spoken to GPs who were told that they needed to demonstrate that they *'reflect more'* and fill in another form to show that they had thought about an educational event *'more deeply'*. Another doctor told me that she was told that unless she filled in a form to prove the *'impact'* of her learning she would not be revalidated (and hence no longer registered with the GMC and no longer able to work as a doctor in the UK).

Is this a proportionate use of time? And what are the harms? A doctor told me about one feedback form which said she was unpleasant and lacked knowledge, despite all the other forms rating her very highly. She implicated this feedback in making her feel insecure and afraid at work, worrying more about who could have said this. One junior doctor, working in a hard-pressed, understaffed speciality had one person write such venomous comments about her (to which she had no right of reply) that she told me *'it was the last straw'*. The data gathered is *'benchmarked'* against other doctors for comparison, but since half of doctors by definition are below average, it's very unclear what the utility is? When I wrote about the appraisal process in the *BMJ*, a typical response was: *'I have loved my job but the pressure of getting all these forms filled in by computer just finished me off. If it wasn't for that I would have kept going for another few years.'*

Of course, had there been good evidence that all these form-fillings made healthcare better and safer it might be worth writing off the time and impact on morale and work capacity. The real hazard of appraisal has been to believe that, as a quality-assurance mechanism, it works. For example, we might expect appraisal to lead to doctors who attract less complaints: since it started, complaints have risen overall.[8] We might have thought that perhaps morale would be improving and high: it is low.[9] We might have thought that perhaps doctors would be keen to stay in posts for as long as possible, and not move abroad or work beyond their expected dates of retiral: GP vacancies are rising and many practices have closed or had to merge.[10] In hospitals the situation is much the same, with rosters of doctors being short-staffed due to *'rota gaps'* – that is, not enough doctors are employed to reliably fill the rota.[11] The effect of complaints on doctors can be profound, with doctors describing symptoms of anxiety, depression and thoughts of suicide, and many doctors describing how it changed them to practice in more risk-adverse ways – *'defensive'* medicine.[12] Tests and treatments can be over-ordered because the doctor is afraid of being found to be *'wrong'* through omission – yet the sins of commission – tests that are full of false positives, treatments of marginal benefit and frequent side effects – are borne by patients.

The problem is manifold. A value had been placed by politicians and managers on gathering and presenting data that is not shared by the professionals who are told to collect and respond to it. The assumption is that doctors are empty vessels, requiring to be filled with the milk and honey of statutory data collection and made to formulaically reflect upon it. But just as it is impossible to enforce a sincere apology, it is impossible to usefully make people think self-critically about their actions when it is done under duress. Instead, it adds to stress, becomes an annoyance and is derided as a cause of problems rather than the solution to them.

Ensuring people are well trained and that the healthcare systems communicate well should be integral to the NHS. But the very integrity of human values in the NHS has been fouled by using these systems to fulfill political ambition rather than patient needs and human values, and in doing so they have culled flexibility and expression. The underlying conflict of targets in this arena – for government compliance versus professional values – should be questioned vigorously.

As for the effect of proliferating complaints – which can now be made to a panoply of organisations – on the workings of the NHS: doctors' description of being *guilty until proven innocent*' in a *'blame business'* should make us question the best ways to ensure safe care as well as taking care of the humans delivering it. The view that *'In cases now, hearsay is more powerful than any other form of evidence ... Innocence just means that we don't yet know what we're guilty of '*. This statement was made by a doctor who is also a regulator of the GMC. Who wants to be treated by a doctor made sick with worry over a complaint? There is nothing worse for safety than an NHS that seeks to apportion blame: *'it may be time to look at the social and economic costs of a wider blame society, to turn blame upon itself, and to change the structure of incentives driving spectacular transparency and the blame business.'* [13]

Top-down IT

At the heart of MTAS was a flawed information technology (IT) system – a catastrophe that cost at least £1.9 million[14] and perhaps as much as £6 million overall.[15]

However, the MTAS fiasco represents pennies down the back of the sofa when compared to the NHS National IT system debacle. Having cost at least £12.4 billion (or more, depending on who you believe), this system was meant to make the NHS paper-free, revolutionise joined-up care and allow patients to choose their own appointments with GPs or hospitals from 2006 onwards. In 2007 the Chair of the Public Accounts Committee said: *'This is the biggest IT project in the world and it is turning into the biggest disaster.'* There had been no cost–benefit analysis in advance.[16] Doctors and nurses who would be using the system hadn't been properly consulted on it.[17] One hospital found that data on patients got *'lost'*, with other clinicians saying *'the software is so clunky, awkward and unaccommodating that we cannot foresee the system working adequately in a clinical context'*.[18] The scheme was disbanded in 2011, but only after even more waste – for example, the early termination of one external IT supplier's contract cost £31.5 million.[19]

Think back to the last time you booked a flight online. How many times did you not realise what box had to be ticked before you could get on to the next screen? How many boxes did you have to tick to locate what you wanted? How many times did the system crash before you got what you wanted? Scotland's NHS decided not to pay for the scheme known as Choose and Book, which started in 2003. This was meant to make GPs in England refer patients *'then and there'* to the hospital they wanted at a time of their choice. Previously, GPs would have referred patients to hospital by dictating or typing a letter at the end of surgery. This new scheme encroached on patient time – either doctors would overrun or doctors would spend less time with patients. It was clumsy and slow, and capable of double-booking appointments.[20] But many GPs were told they must use it. Monitor – in charge of promoting competition, remember – reminded GPs that patients had a *'legal right'* to choose their hospital,[21] and Sir David Nicolson, then Chief Executive of the NHS, told the Public Accounts Committee in 2014 that the way to get GPs to use it was to penalise them for not using it.[22]

Nor did Choose and Book make the referral system better for patients – despite promises that it would decrease the risk of people not attending appointments,[23] it was actually associated with more people not attending.[24] For me this is the head-in-hands moment that exemplifies why we keep getting IT wrong. From the ground up, by listening to what patients and staff need, testing and trialling ideas based on real-world evidence, consensus can build and a system can be developed that is so useful that it will be appreciated. Building a system from the top down, which politicians want and what software developers think patients and staff will need offers strong potential for a wasteful disaster. Indeed, a sociological analysis found descriptions of the technology as being *'inefficient, inflexible, complicated and politically-driven'*, making it unpopular with doctors who knew that their patients would not want to travel 20 or 30 miles to a different hospital. For many people, *'choice'* of hospital was not important – being able to travel only a short distance to a nearer hospital was. One doctor told the researcher: *'We seem to be moving away from curing, caring and comforting to robotic automata.'*[25] In Scotland, the ability to refer by paper was gradually rescinded so that doctors had no option other than to refer via an online referral system[26] (which leaves little space for *'free text'* – contextual information that the doctor on the other end might find helpful) and more tick boxes. One could interpret this system as having been designed to be read by less-well-qualified people or computers, which can only deal in binary yes/no responses. Certainly, it has been found that around one-third of GPs in Scotland never complete the electronic referrals themselves, presumably finding it too burdensome.[27] Incidentally, one of the contractors for this failed NHS IT enterprise in England was Atos, of welfare benefits claim fame. (In Scotland, Atos also has the contract to manage the e-referrals helpdesk.[28])

Clearly, IT is a vital resource with which to organise, track and follow patients, but is the only way top-down? In 2016, the chief executive of the Nuffield Trust felt the need to write that *'strong clinical involvement is needed'* because, *'too many systems have been designed to help the finance department or managers, to reflect what IT specialists think clinicians need, or to satisfy political aspirations.'*

Popular electronic medical records can be created in the NHS. Renal Patient View cost less than £100,000 to set up – even looser down-the-back-of-the-sofa change.[29] It costs a pound or so per patient who opts in; the user can then access all their blood test results and clinic letters – and it is often patients who spot problems with blood results faster than the doctors. Renal Patient View is popular with patients, well used and was designed to enable people to understand their results. It was rolled out to other units stepwise, taking on feedback at each stage. It has grown to be on offer at almost all renal units in the UK. It even has a slot for people to add their own notes, *'what people should know about me'*. It is a gold standard exemplar.[30]

Patients have rightfully rebelled against medicine being done to them rather than for and with them. We are finally appreciating that systems won't work if they are delivered without an understanding or appreciation of the circumstances they are used in. When it comes to clinicians, they are threatened if they do not comply with enforced policy, whether or not it is useful or uses up time that could be put to better use. Instead of clinicians being seen as partners in improvement or having valid reasons for resisting poor systems, they are seen as the problem. This is waste: not simply the cost of developing systems which aren't used, but also the squandering of a massive resource: the professionals committed to the NHS who could have helped.

Referral management

Whether or not Choose and Book is used, when a GP refers a patient to hospital, the patient might reasonably expect that an appointment will follow. Twenty years ago it was common for a consultant to *'vet'* referrals to their clinic – those whom it was thought did or didn't need to be seen urgently could be altered, and occasionally people the consultant didn't feel the need to see would have a letter sent back with advice about what the person was likely to require instead of an appointment.

Enter referral management. How many people know that when they are referred to hospital, that letter may go through a whole management process of its own? It started when data was gathered on which GP practices referred people to hospital. Why did some practices refer more and some refer less? Managers and commissioners saw an opportunity to save money via 'reducing variation' – and, in practical terms, that means cutting the number of referrals being made.

Such a reduction could be a good thing or a bad thing. It could cut down on unnecessary appointments, saving needless trips to hospitals and tests, ensuring that more resources or quicker appointments are then available to people who would actually benefit from them. Or it could delay treatment, sending patients to an inappropriate service, or preventing people from getting care. We surely needed evidence before embarking on another (dis)organisation?

In 2006, it was noted that 'existing systems are viewed as inefficient and it is assumed that technological developments will help improve efficiency' – and 'evidence that the centres are effective is lacking, and costs are difficult to predict' with the 'potential to introduce error and delay'. Crucially, the direction of patients would be under the control of health service managers rather than clinicians: this meant that the GP was no longer the 'gatekeeper' for patients to enter other parts of the NHS.[31] GPs raised concerns that patients' personal information would be shared by staff in the referral centre.[32] Of course, referrals have always been managed or viewed by some hospital staff – it would be impossible to organise appointments otherwise – but by 2011 there was an added complication: some areas were using private companies to run their referral management systems. For example, Hounslow used UnitedHealth[33] and Manchester used Harmoni for several years – a company that rejected or returned 6% of referrals being made.[34] Doctors complained that referrals were rejected on irrelevant criteria and Harmoni's contract was eventually terminated on the grounds of a lack of knowledge of local services (it was run 250 miles away), as well as cost.[35]

Harmoni used podiatrists to triage referrals to vascular specialists. In other areas staff like nurses or physiotherapists, for example, were scrutinising and rejecting referrals.[36] Was this a safe way to manage referrals? Useful? More economical? There had been no randomised controlled trials. This was a policy designed to save money[37] – and in some areas financial incentives were given to practices that could lower their rates of referrals.[38] When the King's Fund reviewed costs, they could find no evidence it had done either.[39]

While electronic letters could automatically transfer some data, they did not improve things in other ways[40] – and I can tell you why: the appointment can easily be over by the time the software has loaded up and done the basics. A systematic review found that peer review and professional support could improve referrals (in other words, allowing doctors to talk and discuss difficult decisions with each other),[41] but referral management schemes were associated with an increase, not the expected decrease, in referrals.[42] Most worryingly, some reports regarded a simple decrease in the number of referrals as a success, without attempting to understand whether the practice was a 'high good' or 'low good' practice – both are absolutely possible (for example, some doctors may have particular expertise in paediatrics or family planning; other doctors may have large numbers of student patients and have less need to refer patients to geriatricians). This scheme did not do what it set out to: the best resource for improving quality was not a highly technological scheme craned in from above, but staff being given the time and space to talk to each other. But how could the scheme have succeeded, when the 'solution' had not been tested before being put into its ill-fitting place?

Some commissioning areas had actually used the Choose and Book system as a supposed opportunity to 'educate' GPs on how to manage the patient without a referral to hospital.

Unsurprisingly, many GPs did not like this and some even abandoned working with the system as a result: '... *clinical buy-in is gained if clinicians are given the power to have significant control over the aims and functioning of the referral management centre (RMC), which in turn means that the RMC's remit meets clinical interests rather more than managerial ones.*'[43] GPs see themselves as working with patients and answerable to them first – not managers.

It is patients we are talking about, not mere players to be moved around an NHS snakes and ladders referral game. And what of the harms? I have had many difficult conversations where a person has been very reluctant to accept a referral. This may have been because of a perception that their needs are not important enough, or because of fear or embarrassment. It is a matter of careful negotiation to agree a plan. I am keen not to oversell what is possible, but neither do I want my patient to endure any more symptoms than necessary. We already know that most referrals come from people living in areas of deprivation,[44] yet there was very limited attention given to the possibility that poorer people would be the ones whose referrals were most likely to be disrupted. The fact that there were no studies into the potential for harm from these schemes is both tragic and simply *'business as usual'*.

Does big data offer better solutions?

As the GP tick-box contract of 2004 appears to be entering a phase of slow demise (albeit decaying faster in Scotland, and due to be replaced entirely), it is likely to be replaced by a podgy morass of other incentives: will these be better or worse?

Parts of the contract have presented practice staff with large datasets; for example, information about how many diazepam tablets are being prescribed, or how many referrals are being made to hospital, or how often people with chronic obstructive airways disease have had to be admitted as an emergency. The data is usually presented in a sliding scale, so that staff can see where they are placed relative to other practices in the area.

Some of this information is quite good. It's fundamentally interesting, and the more nerdish among us can spend many happy hours examining the megabytes of spreadsheets regularly sent to us. The problems arise when unreliable inferences are made about the data. So, for example, part of the contract gathers data about prescribing and then compares it across regions or areas. Some of the data is adjusted to take account of variability in patient groups (for example, a practice with a larger proportion of very old people will be expected to prescribe more drugs for dementia). In Forth Valley there are 150 daily doses of proton pump inhibitors (to reduce stomach acid) per 1,000 patients prescribed compared to 96 in the Highlands.[45] Lanarkshire has 24 daily doses of benzodiazepines per 1,000 patients compared with half that in the Orkney Islands. Of course, we ask: why? Is this to do with the doctors or the patients? Have drug reps been in, pushing their products? Does this represent good prescribing or thoughtless prescribing? For example, to meet the target on antibiotic prescribing, practice prescriptions had to be either in the lower quarter of Scottish practices, or be making reductions in the region of 20%. This could be good, or it could be bad. We know that some antibiotic prescriptions are just unnecessary, such as most childhood ear or throat infections.[46] But antibiotics can also be life-saving. We often use them routinely in the long term to treat acne and, increasingly, to prevent infections for people with severe chronic obstructive airways disease.[47] With these variable uses, it can be hard to know whether a practice's prescribing data represents valid use or inappropriate use. Additionally, there are other drivers that don't necessarily get easily treated with targets – for example, a review of the evidence from Public Health England found that doctor anxiety was a common problem: '*A major factor driving liberal anti-microbial prescribing in primary care is fear due to diagnostic uncertainty and its consequences.*' It also found that: '*The anxiety relates to what might happen to the patient if an antibiotic prescription is not issued – both in clinical terms as well as general dissatisfaction caused by disappointment.*'[48]

This finding is borne out by other big data. A 2015 study found that practices with lower antibiotic-prescribing rates had less satisfied patients.[49] More antibiotic prescribing was linked to higher patient satisfaction scores – and there are financial incentives that encourage GPs to have high satisfaction scores.[50] Various regulators take a keen interest in these scores as supposed *'early warnings'* of poor practice.[51] It's easy to see how GPs working in a fearful environment, afraid of complaints or poor ratings, might be tempted to prescribe more antibiotics than they think necessary. There is a moral tension created by a conflict of interest, but the conflict is not about displeasing one person who wants antibiotics unnecessarily in order to protect the wider community from antibiotic resistance. It is instead a financial conflict of interest, which is entirely avoidable.

Prescribing targets instead link money to doctors making set percentage changes in the levels of prescribing. Is this useful? Are targets actually needed? As usual, there will be unintended consequences. Big data is unprocessed and does not tell us what is a reasonable use and what is not. It does not explain variation, or tell us about quality. And what is *'reasonable'* depends on multiple uncertainties being reconciled by the doctor and patient into a decision of acceptable risk. What is a patient to think if they are not given antibiotics? – that they are not being prescribed because they are not useful, or because the doctor will be financially penalised? Will this undermine trust?

One trial has shown that simply providing the information to doctors about where practices are in prescribing relative to others locally can lead to small but potentially useful reductions in prescribing antibiotics. Perhaps this sort of initiative works because it gives confidence rather then threatens – for there was no financial penalty or incentive involved.[52] This study – in a similar fashion to the prescribing targets – did not assess whether or not the prescriptions were good quality or not. I would argue, however, that an incentive-free scheme is less likely to create systematic under-

or overprescribing of antibiotics. Similarly, it is nonsense to insist that practices which are already low prescribers for some drugs should reduce still further regardless of whether this is good for patients or not. Yet it is business as usual when it comes to prescribing incentives for GPs. Prescribing should rely on professional and patient values and judgement – and if that judgement can be supported by careful consideration of where one lies in the bigger prescribing picture, excellent.

The price of quality control

At the heart of this way of thinking, there is an assumption that the NHS cannot improve without financial incentives, and that forced targets are a better means to that end than co-operative and evidence-based systems.

In England, the Care Quality Commission (CQC) was formed in 2009 by combining three old regulators. The CQC was to cover both health and social care, but with less money. Old regulation was paid for (in the main) by government: new regulation was to be paid for by those being regulated.[53] For a typical GP practice this has increased from £725 to £4,839; if a surgery has a 'branch' (the same doctor working on a rota at a smaller base than the main surgery, which often happens in rural or deprived areas), the surgery would have to pay two sets of fees.[54] Perhaps all this would be worth it, though, if inspection was leading to better care for patients? After all, the Department of Health has said: '*These fees allow CQC's tough inspection regime to drive up standards across the country.*' [55]

The CQC decided to inspect practices by using so-called '*intelligent monitoring*', which involves using the available data – such as that from the GP contract and the patient survey – to identify those practices having an '*elevated risk*' or not.[56] This was widely publicised in the press, with many local newspapers reporting practices as '*high risk*' or having the '*worst doctors*'.[57] But when the CQC went to make a visit to the practices they declared were at '*elevated risk*', there was found to be a very poor relationship between this risk grading and those practices later found to be '*inadequate*'. Data had been wrongly entered, despite this flaw being pointed out to the CQC,[58] which was forced to withdraw the scheme and apologise.[59] For most GPs, finding one's name and photograph on the front page of a newspaper story critical of the practice was deeply shaming. One doctor I spoke to said that it made her want to run away: *'I've never experienced anything like it.'*

So, *'intelligent monitoring'* delivered errors and judgemental language. The contract – for £1.5 million – to supply this *'intelligence'* was won by McKinsey. Pre-tender, McKinsey were granted exclusive access to data – something that was against public procurement rules.[60] And where was the evidence that *'intelligent monitoring'* was capable of detecting the allegedly dangerous practices? Of course, there wasn't any: there had been no meaningful pilots, no trial. The CQC went on to spend much time trawling websites for comments about practices – when, surely, it would possess the knowledge that self-selecting commentators[61] are unlikely to create a fair representation; this is a problem that even professional polling companies get wrong,[62] and it all amounts to an absurd waste of money.

And there were human costs too. Dr Martin Brunet – who I know personally – is the sort of kind, careful, intelligent and wise person that anyone would be glad to have as their GP. He wrote about the process of the CQC coming to inspect his practice: *'It is infantilising and humiliating as two officious inspectors have free rein to poke around your beloved practice, ignorant of your unique ethos and values, careless of your history or the joys and challenges of serving your unique patient population. There is no attempt to celebrate what you do well, just a begrudging acknowledgement that may appear somewhere in the report, but will in no way compensate for your more obvious failings.'*

The practice was criticised for not having photographs of the staff on file. This may be useful in a massive organisation but in an ordinary general practice, where the staff are also your friends and the length of time someone has worked beside you is measured in decades and not days, this is patently unnecessary. Having rolls of paper (used to cover examination couches) kept on the floor was not acceptable (even though there is no infection risk from doing so).[63]

The experience of inspection reads to me like institutional bullying. Brunet writes, *'Take patient safety, for example. Naïve, foolish doctor that I am, I thought it might have something to do with staying up to date, giving my patients time to explain their problems, examining them carefully and seeing them promptly in an emergency.'* He is, of course, not the only doctor to report an inspection as a humiliation.

Dr Dominique Thomson, who had worked in a student health service, described the attitude during her inspection: *'It was the worst day of my career and the most negative, most undermining, most demoralising experience of my life ... From the moment the inspectors walked through the door, they were nitpicky, negative and pedantic, and not in a helpful way. It was as if they were unable to see anything positive at any stage.'* Her staff were told they were not caring, despite no evidence to back this up. Another practice manager, so traumatised by the inferences made, handed in her resignation.[64]

These experiences arise from several cultural clashes. The values of inspectors (in favour of filing, paperwork and rigid protocol over evidence) do not match those of practice staff (a preference for continuity of care, time with patients, experience and pragmatism, topped with vocation which forms a large part of personal identity). A top-down data-driven desire for uniformity finds itself at odds with grassroots experience. No one involved wants to see substandard practices, care homes or hospitals, and I do not think there is any desire not to be regulated – it is a question of evidence, focus and opportunity costs. Preparation for inspection, too, takes most practices at least 20 hours, and appointments have to be cancelled to fit in meetings with the visiting CQC.[65]

The chief inspector of GPs has said that some surgeries don't self-acclaim enough, resulting in them failing to be highly rated[66] – marketing yourself to your regulator seems highly prized in the post-HSCA NHS era. When the CQC launched its expensive, non-evidenced *'intelligent monitoring'* it did so in the wake of the Francis Report, and as such it looks to me like a keenness to be doing *'something'* regardlesss of whether it was useful or not. The CQC itself was heavily criticised for not picking up systemic problems in Morecambe Bay hospital. The Francis Report even stated that *'current outcomes are overly bureaucratic and fail to separate clearly what is absolutely essential from that which is merely desirable'.* Indeed, the CQC had tried to suppress a report that found it had failed to detect poor care at Morecambe Bay hospital.[67]

In some ways I have sympathy for the CQC. It's clear that quality is hard to measure: much is subjective and will be judged differently depending on the individuals doing the judging. Yet the CQC has chosen to grade services as *'inadequate', 'good'* or *'outstanding',* without realising the problems this creates. Sure, there are plain features of quality, such as being able to see a doctor in good time when ill, or having records kept confidentially. But it would be far better for the CQC to ensure that everyone is getting *'good enough'* care, and to use transparency and professional values to ensure that services continue to improve. In 2013, even the chair of the CQC said that the organisation could not improve quality, and this would be the job of people on the ground: *'We should remain sceptical about what a regulator can do.'* [68]

The resultant harms are not just about demoralised staff, but the creation of fear and resentment. Who becomes more likely to speak up about poor care when the consequences of doing so may end careers and leave doctors with *'serious psychological damage, even to the extent of suicidal depression'?* [69]

Of course, if multiple hospitals are *'failing'* their CQC inspections perhaps this has a bigger meaning. Maybe it becomes impossible to provide decent and safe care when staff and services are being cut because of a shrinking budget? We should not be spending money evaluating the failure of services to provide the impossible, but putting the money to better use through direct, hands-on care.

Much of what happens is invidious. A hospital which

manages to treat all its patients within nine or 12 months rather than 18 may be told that such an 'overperformance' means it has been getting too much money and therefore can manage with less next year. By contrast, hospitals with long waiting lists and times may be rewarded with extra money to bail them out – even though the root of the problem may be poor ways of working rather than a lack of funding. 'The NHS has to move from a culture where it bails out failure to one where it rewards success.'[70] Failure is seen as something that can be mitigated for and controlled internally.[71]

In Scotland, there is a different organisation called Healthcare Improvement Scotland, which does the same kind of work as the CQC. It is not perfect. But it runs on an understanding of assumed co-operation. Visits from staff tend to be low-key, discursive and formative. Its reports highlight good practice and recommend what could improve, and the tone is essentially non-confrontational.[72] I know healthcare workers who choose to take part in inspecting other practices, because: 'I like to see what others are doing and I can learn from them and bring that back here.' Indeed, there is much research that finds 'peer audit and feedback as well as mutual support by colleagues are crucial in inducing change'.[73] In Scotland there is not the fear and angst that my colleagues in England endure. The cultures of regulation can rule through bottom-up support that encourages and draws on professional values ('we all like to feel our practices are the best practice'[74]) or by attempting top-down imposition, creating conflict, fear, a loss of faith and, ultimately, frustrated refusals to engage.

Interview

Colm O'Mahony, consultant in sexual health

I've been a consultant in genito-urinary medicine in Chester since 1990. We used to have a fantastic service. We had a dozen compliments from patients a week – were treasured by GPs and hospital staff (especially emergency medicine). Staff were happy and enthusiastic; it was a great place to work. Then the Health and Social Care Act happened. Within a year, we had a total disaster. We don't know why, but sexual health services were moved out of the NHS contract system and we were contracted by councils instead. So now the council were in charge of bins, potholes and sexual health. The council knew nothing about sexual health.

The contract went out to tender. So we had to go through a tendering process. I met people I'd never met before – the Trust procurement team, finance officers, managers, commissioners, public health staff. We spent a good nine months writing our bid. Most of this was done by clinical colleagues and myself, at the end of the clinical day. I was confident we would retain the contract. I had been the expert consultant on a sexual health tender panel previously, so knew the system and process. Alarm bells should have rung though, when I heard the council were not going to hold interviews for a £12.5 million contract. The contract was awarded to East Cheshire Trust (ECT) based in Macclesfield, 50 miles away. We asked for explanations – who was on the panel that made the decision? They refused to tell us, but FOI forced the admission that there was no doctor on the panel and even worse no one who had ever worked in a sexual health clinic! The council had said that £2.5million per annum was the maximum amount available, but, surprisingly, the winning bid was £2.8million. We appealed; the council reluctantly ran the process again, this time adding a GP, who had once worked in an STD clinic ten years ago, to the panel! Can you imagine a surgical tender being assessed with the only expert being someone who had once been a junior doctor in surgery? We spent about two days a week for three months rewriting our bid. But the decision stayed the same. No details of how the decision was made have been given – due to 'commercial confidentiality'. I appealed to the local government ombudsman (LGO) but after months was told that I hadn't 'suffered enough personal injustice' for the LGO to investigate.

I'm still not sure why they won. Their bid was put together by a tender-management person and a senior nurse. There was no sexual health consultant input into their bid. We know their service model proposed a mobile clinic that would move every six months! This brought back memories of the old portakabin days we used to put up with, 30 years ago. From a freedom of information request we know they and the council spent months trying to set up a modular building in the car park of a sports centre. When this 'innovative' idea proved impossible they moved us – for many of the staff ended up being subcontracted to work there – from the huge clinic at the hospital into a few rooms in a GP complex in the town centre. We don't have enough space. We have no appointments for a week – a week! Before, 100% of our patients would have had an appointment in 48 hours. A sexual health service in a big city and no appointments for a week! – it's horrendous. Even worse, it's so packed that patients just turn up and wait. One Saturday, before we opened, there was a queue outside the building – right underneath the big, garish sign saying 'sexual health clinic'. Just imagine the embarrassment as the 'Big Red Chester Tour Bus' drove slowly past. One patient told me a 'white van man' pulled up and leered at the queue. It was just awful. I went outside myself and tore off the sign. Ironically, after months of receiving relentless complaints, this generated the first compliment the clinic ever had, one young patient wrote: 'I'm glad that dreadful garish sign has been removed.'

We used to have close connections with other disciplines in the hospital – we used to be adjacent to A&E at the Countess Hospital. So we could see patients with herpes right away, look at rashes they were concerned about, be immediately available *if any of our HIV patients ended up in A&E. Doctors from the hospital used to sit in with us to learn. We went to grand rounds, we talked to our consultant colleagues and we were involved in teaching and training. It means that a huge hospital like the Countess has no sexual health service. Many of our staff have left. Our team has been broken up – between HIV, which is still based in the hospital intermittently, and sexual health based in the GP complex. Now pregnant women, with antenatal bloods positive for syphilis or Hep B have to travel into town to see us in the GP centre. It's no longer a seamless service.*

Of course, I have been tempted to retire. It's so sad. All of this could have been avoided. Hundreds of thousands of pounds and how much time has been wasted? Nothing good has come of it – nothing. I now go to contract meetings, and managers and public health are talking about 'key performance indicators' related to trivia but no one seems appalled at the fact that access is now awful – there are no appointments!

It was all much simpler years ago, when we were just contracted by the Primary Care Trust to run the service. There was no hassle with managers or from finance, we were a treasured part of the hospital Trust. We just got on with it. I don't blame East Cheshire Trust at Macclesfield for this. It's not their fault they won the tender. They will never admit it, but I suspect they were more surprised to win it than we were to lose it! Of course I'm working closely with my new 'boss' to make the best of this mess. ECT are as keen as me and my staff to make this better and get back to providing a service as good as what we used to have. At least it's an NHS Trust, so more focused on quality than profit. This process – through the HSCA – has caused pointless, untold damage to sexual health services throughout England.

Finally, I hadn't expected this interview to be anything other than me calmly reflecting on what had happened to the service, so I was not prepared for the reawakening of the anger, frustration and intense sense of injustice that I thought I had gotten over – obviously not.

8

Professionals and Patients: The Human Capital of the NHS

William Osler, the Canadian physician who died in 1919, has retained the admiration and respect of subsequent generations of doctors. Many of his writings are pithily contemporaneous, including his classic 1910 essay *Aequanimitas*, in which he declared: *'The practice of medicine is an art, not a trade; a calling, not a business; a calling in which your heart will be exercised equally with your head.'*[1] Just as doctors Hill and Bourne debated whether professional, ethical medicine could exist in an environment where financial profit was the master, Osler was calling attention to vocation in medicine. This, he argued, is not a business created for entrants to grow rich at the expense of patients, but a deeper matter of moral appeal. Yet the workings of the NHS have, for general practitioners in particular, clawed at the rationale of doctors' decision-making and left patients questioning the motivation for their doctors' activities. Does vocation in medicine still hold true? Are financial incentives useful, and, if so, what are their side effects? Do they benefit patients as much as doctors, or are they a mechanism for political control rather than for quality care for patients?

Should the treatment of illness be bound by the rules of the market – with its flexible factors of supply, demand and price – so that the availability of medical treatment becomes determined by an individual's ability to meet the cost? Or should medicine be thought of as a vocation, driven by ideals and harnessing dedication, not just intellect? This book has argued that markets in medicine have been serially flawed, and the preceding chapters have shown how the reforms to the

NHS have wasted time, money and effort, focusing on things of little value to patients, creating disruption and diverting effort into meeting harmful targets which do not result in safer, better healthcare. These market-based reforms create instability and waste resources in top-down administration; they are collectively bad for us.

Are markets the only option? Of course not. Something fundamental has been missing from the equation: the staff who work in it and the patients, their carers and families who use it. Together, these people are the biggest resource the NHS has. Healthcare staff do not go into service as empty and recalcitrant vessels, waiting to be filled with protocols and instructions set down for them by remote committees, working only when chided or rewarded, financially or otherwise. Healthcare workers often have long training periods, which they have been allowed to embark on after a competitive process in which they will have demonstrated their wish to go beyond the mere *tasks* and subsume the values and ethical standards of a professional.

The most celebrated physician of the Roman empire, Greek physician and philosopher Galen, told us that good doctors must *'despise money and cultivate temperance in order to stay the course'*.[2] In 1911, a doctor wrote in to the *Lancet* to declare: *'More and more are we urged to consider the fact that all the practice of medicine is a business, in that it is a means of livelihood, and that consequently it ought to be conducted on business methods ... Yet is it undoubtedly the case that in all times the highest and worthiest thought in medicine has considered that there is a fundamental and unbridgeable chasm between the practice of the healing art and all commercial pursuits of whatever kind ... the customs of the commercial world, worthy of respect though they may be at the hands of the commercial man, are based upon first principles essentially different from those upon which the practice of the healing art has been from time immemorial established.'* [3]

When the NHS was created, GPs were not made salaried like consultants. Instead they became independent contractors to the new NHS. This left them competing against each other, with poorer areas being under-doctored relative to richer neighbourhoods.

One GP wrote to the *Lancet* in 1947: '*Almost anyone can write a prescription copied from the National Formulary, and fill in a form or send a patient to hospital. It is quantity that counts today, not quality. How much better if this cut-throat competition, so beloved by the BMA, had been entirely eliminated by paying us a salary compatible with our experience and years of practice. Happy indeed are those young and healthy enough to emigrate.*'[4]

These words could just as easily be written in 2016 as we administer '*Friends and Family tests*' or publish CQC ratings, supposedly to drive up competition to be '*the best*'.

Motivations: missionary zeal or monetary reward?

Historian Dr Graham Smith has amusingly categorised GPs in the 1960s as belonging to camps of '*socialists, businessmen and missionaries*'.[5] He has a serious point. There have always been doctors with missionary zeal, and who have acted – with religiosity or without – as though their work was a ministry. The socialists believed that health inequalities were a scourge on both the rich and poor, and that outlook was exemplified by GP Julian Tudor Hart, who worked in the Welsh valleys in the belief that universal free healthcare was only fair and morally right care.[6] As he put it: '*Where health care providers compete on a commodity market, their natural tendency is to magnify their own skills and ignore those of their patients, and to maximise sales without regard to social or even biological need.*'[7]

But it is the business folk who have been most well catered for in the most recent incarnations of the NHS, even though, as discussed in Chapter 6, a health marketplace, rife with competition and profit-seeking, is deeply problematic. Indeed, there is much evidence of the harms of treating healthcare as a commodity instead of as a resource. The best example of the appalling and harmful lure of markets in medicine is the private sector in '*health screening*' marketed at healthy people, as touched on in Chapter 4 (and discussed in *The Patient*

Paradox). For here, people are routinely exposed to expensive interventions of no medical value and even of harm. Many private clinics offer heavily advertised *'MOT'* services, including scans, blood tests and ECG tests – but these are not proven to benefit people; instead they create multiple false positives, which are often passed back to the NHS to be dealt with. As a GP there are few things quite so frustrating as being passed a 20-page medical report for my opinion – a cost the NHS is simply meant to absorb while the private sector makes a tidy profit and walks away. In the meantime, I have to use further NHS appointments to deliver the reassurance that was promised by the private sector but which it failed to deliver. IVF clinics in the private sector use league tables and *'success'* rates, which are made available to the public, as advertising. Fertility clinics can boost their standing in these tables by generating multiple births. However, twin, triplet or quad pregnancies are more risky for both the babies and the mother, increasing the risk of premature birth or the need for operative delivery. They also significantly impact on the NHS resources that are needed, whether in terms of labour and birth or cribs in neonatal units.[8] The private sector has also been found to have inherent biases: for example, the fee-per-service model means that there is an increased risk of children being exposed to tonsillectomy in the private sector compared with the NHS.[9] The impact any of this might have on follow-up care in the NHS is not met by the private sector, which simply washes its hands.

As a junior doctor I would sometimes wonder where certain consultants were, only to be told that they were *'down the mint'* – that is, working from the private hospital and unavailable to the NHS patients they were meant to be responsible for. I was present years ago when a moribund patient – milky pale, hardly breathing, and with no measurable blood pressure – was stretchered into our medical unit direct from the private hospital where she had had complications from surgery and they were unable to deal with it. She needed equipment and expertise that was not available in the luxury hospital she had paid for: it is a dirty little secret that some private hospitals have minimal, and often only basically qualified, medical staff on duty overnight. And, of course, any resultant death would be recorded as occurring in the NHS failing despite the fact that it was not responsible for the circumstances that had led to 'complications'.

These anecdotes represent merely the tip of the iceberg of harms done by the medical model as a business. In 1980 the campaign group Radical Statistics found that elective operations to remove piles and tonsils varied internationally according to how doctors were paid. More fees per item of service meant more surgery, even when these were more invasive operations for breast cancer or hysterectomies. The difference was the presence of money as a motivator: '... *apart from the questionable morality inherent in attempting to bias professional practice through appealing to avarice, this system has further distasteful potential: for example, doctors may employ salaried personnel (especially nurses) to perform procedures while they pocket the fees.*' [10]

Money was used as a motivator in the GP contract of 1994 – paid by the Department of Health to produce behavioural change in doctors it deemed to be 'good'. But these were not behavioural changes that were necessarily evidence-based or good for patients. Should GPs ever have accepted money for adopting the Choose and Book method, which only propagated the internal NHS market? Could Galen have dreamt that the doctors who followed after him would be paid per diagnosis of dementia?

But money is not the only motivator. What of that old-fashioned, slightly embarrassing admission – vocation? It is what prospective medical students are quizzed about the presence of, and what junior doctor training schemes for general practice are still called. There are claims that medical vocation no longer exists, most famously in recent years by Jeremy Hunt, who told the BBC in 2015 that he wanted '*that sense of vocation and professionalism brought back into the contract*'.[11] Galen went even further: he believed that doctors '*cannot be hard working if one is continually drinking or eating or indulging in sex*'. Galen's expectations of vocational practice border on the monastic.[12]

Bevan told his colleagues that he persuaded consultants to join the NHS in 1948 only because he was '*stuffing their mouths with gold*'.[13] In 2012, Christine Odone asked in the *Daily Telegraph*: '*Does a doctor have a profession or a vocation?... the doctors who propose to strike over cuts to their pension pots make it clear that they look on their work as a nice little earner – the average GP earns £110,000 a year – rather than a whole-hearted vocation.*' She went on, '*why should a good doctor be afraid of competition? And why should the mediocre and plainly bad ones be exempt from it, when the rest of us ordinary mortals must compete in everything we do?*' [14] Doctors, in her view, should be both fully vocational but also keenly competing in a medical marketplace.

In 1967 *A Fortunate Man* by John Berger was published, about general practice in the 1960s. This portrait of the working life of general practitioner John Sassall is now regarded as a classic. Berger writes: '*The doctor is the familiar of death. When we call for a doctor, we are asking him to cure us and to relieve our suffering, but, if he cannot cure us, we are also asking him to witness our dying. The value of the witness is that he has seen others die. He is the intermediary between us and the multitudinous dead. He belongs to us and he has belonged to them. And the hard but real comfort which they offer through him is still that of fraternity ... The function of fraternity is recognition.*' [15]

How do we monetise that, place it in a '*quality framework*' and prove that this '*works*'? People do not come to see a doctor to discuss a straightforward symptom but because of '*upsetting events, social isolation, psychiatric disorder, and desire for health information*'.[16] In my experience as a doctor, I know that dealing with death is not just crucial to serve the community, but is also the source of profound professional fulfilment. It is what I have been trained for, both by textbook and by watching and learning from others. If done well enough it will also give comfort to the families and friends who live on. This reveals itself in the conversations had with relatives five or ten years later, or in a chance meeting in the supermarket. Then there is the door handle moment, when a patient goes to leave but hesitates: *'Can I just ask you about...'* It is, of course, the real reason the person came, concerning the worry about something – possibly seemingly minor – that has been eating into sleep and terrorising wakefulness, and which the good GP will deal with. This will be of huge value to the person but may irritate the next waiting patient who writes a scathing online review of their late-running GP. It is just as Professor Arrow has written: we only get full information in retrospect, and sometimes never.

In 1991, GP David Widgery wrote decrying the practice of modern medicine, detached from human meaning: *'The New Model GP is hunched over the computer screen calculating uptake and turnover, auditing not clinical skill but fiscal returns and acting as an accountant, an architect, a travel agent, a manager: almost anything but a doctor.'* [17] But earlier in his book he wrote of something else: joy. He made a visit to newborn twins, born after a difficult conception and pregnancy: *'I wanted to cry because words, even "joy" and "happiness" seemed so hopelessly inexpressive.'* Here there is none of that numb industrial, tick-box medicine by rote, of being a doctor who is only a cardboard cut-out of medicine, of being merely a bystander without the means to be of use. Instead, he describes the raw, muscular reality of pain and joy, and death and life. There is the binding of self to vocation, with all the human value that brings.

Happinesss in work is still possible, oxymoronic as that might sound while, as I write, the junior doctors' contract is being imposed. I love my work, despite the stresses and frustrations, and I am not alone. Doctors in Australia, working in deprived areas, report finding *'meaning and satisfaction'* in a job they *'love'* in work that was the *'right thing to do'*.[18] This attitude is neither fluffily or saintly altruistic but a description of genuine fulfilment and intellectual challenge not readily found elsewhere. Iona Heath, a former president of the

Royal College of GPs, writes of the *'love of ordinary general practice'*.[19] One doctor talked of how a patient had *'taught me to be grateful with what you have in life ... There's very very good people out there that deal with a lot in life and if you can facilitate them in any way, well that's your job – that's all you're doing'*. Or simply: *'... it also meets needs that I have as a human ... to feel that I belong and that I am valued.'* [20]

A woman brought up in the care system described how she is still *'wary of health professionals'*, but because her general practitioner encouraged her to keep coming back to see her as needed: *'That way I don't always have to refer to my history of abuse or repeatedly tell someone that I don't know about my birth family's medical history ... she never judges my decisions. She simply tells me about the pros and cons and encourages me to think about it for the future. She is always smiling and looks at me when I'm talking so I always feel able to ask her even "silly" questions.'* [21]

Instead, the values of general practice have not been captured in the way the speciality has been recently organised or paid; and as a consequence, those values have been rent invisible to many outsiders. GP David Zigmund writes:

'General practice was never the most glamorous or charismatic of medical specialties, but for many decades its better forms commanded much vocational loyalty and enduring personal contentment. The basis for such quiet and stable satisfaction lay in its human relationships: GPs' consultations took place almost entirely between the doctor and patient, and could then sensitively extend to the patient's primary relationships. Forty years ago this was aptly called "family doctoring". Other agencies were little involved, and then usually only by invitation. Because there was so little intrusion or management from elsewhere, personal understandings, and then affections, could flourish. Such human engagements have been changed utterly... The increasingly fatigued and stressed GP becomes torn between his need to obey governance and the wish to create good human sense and connection with this person now. Increasing our mandatory tasks of obedience and administration has crippled

our better human capacities and responses... our profession has become humanity-famined.[22]

Medicine itself requires human relationships at its heart, for the benefit of both patients and doctors. So how can we think that the values of the market – efficiency, competition, tendering and legal contracts – will not interfere with the humane values of support and vocation?

The humanitarian values in medicine are under threat because of the way we are expected to work. That is the danger that gives me most concern. Just as in Osler's day, applicants to medical school are expected to describe their vocation. There is no shortage of bright, committed people who want to work in healthcare. Yet the structure of the NHS means that these vocational values are constantly being pressed under continual and systematic challenge to their expression. While doctors accept, as the GMC says, that they should always act in patients' *'best interests',* we would not expect very human doctors to be immune from financial incentives to prescribe a less good drug or operation in order to make more profit. If a rich person with a minor injury was treated in A&E before a poor person with a life-threatening injury, we would be outraged because we expect doctors to treat according to need. But need is not always explicit. Nor is there debate about the purposes of medicine. The market structure infers that is possible to make efficiencies, and those efficiencies make profit, which then becomes the motivation to act. Alternatively, the market works by expanding its reach – and in medicine, that reach can extend into procedures which do not benefit patients, only doctors' profit margins. On the other hand, vocationally driven healthcare speaks of an ongoing professional responsibility where the values are in the relationships. Philosopher Michael Sandler writes: *'The era of market triumphalism has coincided with a time when public discourse has been largely empty of moral and spiritual substance.'*[23] Are we too afraid to talk about motivators other than money, such as pride, satisfaction and the pleasure to be had in doing good work?

General practitioners have been treated by government as barriers to care, perceived to be motivated primarily by money, not facilitators of professional skills and values. Recurrent reforms from the 1990s onwards have been predicated on the belief that money is the best motivator for change. This has resulted in too much medicine – treatment by rote rather than because it matters to you, the individual patient. The seams of vocation and ethics are pulled at by incentives which request compliance, not the interrogation of suitability for the individual.

Fellowship fractured

Professionals may be well qualified people but they are still human, with all the flaws that entails, rather than robots, completing tasks to order. This humanness, together with vocational and professional practice, is a strength. We know that having continuity of care with the same staff leads to better quality of care and is valued by patients, especially people who are vulnerable,[24] or who have long-term conditions[25] or need care across many different venues.[26] Continuity is about responsibility: a moral contract to a long-term relationship, where staff take responsibility not just for the moment in hand, but for helping with the information patients and families need for future planning. And then there is the emotional connection and support: *'I felt somebody really cares about me,'* said one patient.[27]

For anyone who has been ill, it's easy to identify with the trust in other humans that is necessary when we are not able to think as clearly or research the evidence on our condition for ourselves. Healthcare staff were more motivated to wash their hands when reminded by signs that it could prevent disease in patients compared to signs saying they could prevent disease in themselves.[28] So don't we have to accept this evidence and ensure that the system we place NHS staff into recognises and uses their vocational motivation to the utmost while helping to eliminate the human failures we are all prone to?

In their remarkable book *Intelligent Kindness*, John Ballatt and Penelope Campling explain and explore the moral contract between medicine and society.[29] Campling has written: *'It is easy to forget the appalling nature of some of the jobs carried out by healthcare staff day in, day out – the damage, the pain, the mess they encounter, the sheer stench of diseased human flesh and its waste products. Contact with emotional distress and disturbance can be equally, if not more, harrowing. Existential questions about identity, suffering, madness and death are raised and may put people in touch with extreme feelings of confusion, pain and loss.'* [30]

She describes how feeling part of a team acts as a buffer to the stresses of work, but that the team is often broken down and unclear. Just as staff without close bonds with workmates do less well, so *'patients often complain that they see a series of junior doctors and do not know the name of their consultant'.* Change has been aggressively promoted in the NHS, yet, say Ballatt and Campling, *'it is the uncritical promotion of constant change and imposition of new ideologies that is the main social defence system in the modern health service, overloading and fragmenting the system and distracting from the task of caring for the sick and dying'.* Critics of reform are usually criticised themselves (as being *'out of date'* or *'unfair'*[31]), but there seems to have been little public discourse on how reforms have affected the unwritten infrastructure of the NHS – that is, the knitting of professional teams and their patients. A well-resourced staff, capable of supporting itself, will serve patients far better than a stressed, depleted team. Yet the construction and capabilities of teams – for creating safety and good care in the NHS – have been given scant attention.

Where staff report better health and wellbeing themselves, the care experienced by patients is generally reported as better. Teams work well together when they know each other: *'Organisations also need to focus on developing cultures that are person centred – not just task focused – by valuing and building on the excellent care and commitment delivered by many staff throughout the NHS.*[32] And teamworking itself is associated with better staff mental health.[33] Although the research states that teams working across disparate physical locations will find it harder to work closely, care has not been organised to reflect this. The reality of community care where I work is that our health visitors and district nurses have been removed from being based at our practice – where they had coffee mugs and we could informally exchange information several times a day – to a central clinic miles away. Instead of knocking at a door to work out how best to look after a dying patient together, we have been asked to use a call centre. It is not just communicating messages and organising care that we need our colleagues for. It is also, crucially, to them that we normally turn to discuss difficult problems, when we are questioning our judgement and wondering if we should or could do anything differently. Is this not 'safety'? How can a team knit together when they have been deliberately and repeatedly disjointed? It is especially important to consider this in light of the fact that the NHS has been ordered into reorganisation after re-disorganisation. The build up and fracturing of team cohesion and spirit has been uncosted, both in financial terms and in relation to the 'added value' that the relationships themselves generate.

No wonder that British general practitioners are highly stressed, with the shortest consultation times and highest stress levels out of 11 comparable countries investigated by the Commonwealth Fund. The stress is mirrored in their plummeting job satisfaction in the last five years.[34] 'Our public model of the ideal professional care-giver is of someone who can be endlessly human to others without needing anything human in return,' wrote two mental health practitioners in the Guardian. 'By pursuing target-driven and finance-driven policies that take no account of the mind of the carer, successive governments have succeeded only in ratcheting up the emotional burden on professionals.' As sick leave goes up, the healthcare team only become more stressed themselves.[35] In turn, patients do not get as good care as they should: consequently, professional satisfaction in doing good work declines, and the humane value of the work disintegrates.

Our institutions pay scant attention to the system problems that contribute to avoidable stress, such as electronic medical records, where higher use of them is associated with burnout of doctors,[36] or complaints processes. As politicians promote a consumer culture rather than a partnership of collaboration, complaints to the NHS have accelerated.[37] The process of investigating and concluding a complaint is frequently long, drawn out and often described by doctors as humiliating. Between 2005 and 2013, 28 doctors died by suicide while under investigation by the GMC. One of the recommendations an independent review made to the GMC was that medical students should have 'emotional resilience training'.[38] But what about tackling the underlying problems of why work is so stressful? Why are so many complaints being made against doctors, increasing their risk of self-harm and suicide?[39] The staff in the NHS are its biggest asset, but cannot be worked as though they are angels, practicing magic with invisible resources, and be emotionally resilient enough to be unaffected by complaints – while caring as only humans can.

Stresses and strains

The NHS, far from being a paragon of a healthy working environment, is often a challenging and uncomfortable place to work.

As far back as 1960 it was known that stress and anxiety were common features of nursing. If a nurse was devastated at making a mistake she was 'usually reprimanded instead of being helped'. One described how 'you must reprimand someone, even if you don't know who really did it'. Mature, deep-thinking nurses were more likely to leave the profession.[40] The emotion of work is reflected in staff: the more professionals care for their dying patients, the more they experience feelings of loss.[41] Emotional exhaustion, burnout and 'depersonalisation' is very common among clinicians who respond to surveys.[42] What are the causes of such overwhelming stress, and why is it such an intractable problem? In response to the suicide of a general practitioner friend, one doctor wrote: 'Primary care has become dramatically more complex and demanding in under a decade. There has been a deliberate, cynical shifting of workload *from secondary to primary care without an accompanying shift of resources and without relevant professional support, training, and development: we are just expected to "get on with it".* There is longstanding evidence that NHS staff suffer high amounts of distress:[43] there is also evidence that more distressed staff are less happy with the work they do and the more likely to work in hospitals with less good outcomes.[44]

At the same time, expectations of what the NHS can provide have altered among the general public: *'We now have a more consumerist, demand-driven society that talks about rights but says little about responsibility and, in many areas, treats the NHS as though it were a 24-hour supermarket or take-away outlet. This is coupled with the explicit encouragement (often by health managers no less) for the public to complain about services and an increasingly irresponsible legal profession which has fuelled a culture of litigation against doctors on a "no win, no fee" basis.'*[45]

How did doctors and patients get so far apart? How did we end up in opposition, as if observing the other as the enemy? One of the earliest lessons I learned, from my ancient *Oxford Handbook of Clinical Medicine,*[46] was that patients were not the opposition or your hindrance, and not simply the recipients of my efforts either. Have a cup of tea with a patient, the authors suggested, take a break and have a chat, and you will be rewarded: *'... patients are sources of renewal, not just devourers of your energies.'* Although the hours were horrible, there was the sense of teamship, surrounding and supporting. It included patients and their families, who were appreciative of our efforts. It was a patient, decades ago, who pointed out to me that the drug I was about to give him was wrong – and he was (to my great relief) not angry with me, but pleased to have helped (and triggered a review of the way drugs were stored). I was knackered, but had a sense of fulfilment. As one paediatrician has written, on the elusive nature of *'life–work balance'*: *'...the border between life and work vanished, work became life, and life became work. We all have some better and some worse days, but as physicians by the end of each day we*

will have made a difference in at least one child's life ... Two
children died last night during my call in the ICU. One family
saved the lives of four children by donating their son's organs.
The other family told my team what an honour it was for them
to meet us and they will never forget how we helped them cope
with the tragic death of their 12-year-old daughter. I am tired,
exhausted, and hungry. But right now, I am balanced.' [47]

This story illustrates vocation in action. Junior doctors now
have little cohesive team structure; they work erratic shifts
often reflecting a lack of care for them and their sleep patterns.
They have little control over their working lives, unable to
even know when they can get married.[48] Many junior doctors'
rotas are chronically underfilled, meaning that they asked or
ordered to fill 'rota gaps'[49] beyond their already long contracted
hours. Bizarrely, just as the imposition of their contract was
announced by the health secretary, so was a review into why
morale among junior doctors is so low[50] – a juxtaposition that
would have been laughable were it not reality. Being treated
badly does not make for loyalty among staff or breed goodwill,
joy or pleasure in the workplace.

Listen to the patients ...

If health professionals bring their own motivation and desire
to do a good job, is that enough? No: and it does not need to
be. Patients, as I have already said, can be *'sources of renewal'*. I
have kept all the thank-you cards I have received in my career,
and they are utterly sustaining – but if the NHS really is for the
citizens, patients and families, they need integral involvement.

Twenty or 30 years ago, it was *'doctor knows best'* and good
patients asked no difficult questions and swallowed the tablets
they had been ordered to. This is, of course, appalling. My
outrage at the advertising masquerading as information for
private screening tests was what kickstarted my writing career.
People are capable of making well-informed choices, I wrote,
to anyone who would listen, but we need good information
to do so. There is a moral responsibility for doctors to uphold
patient autonomy and choice.

Choice, though, is not enough. For decades, researchers have been investigating many things that simply don't matter to patients. Now, sure, researchers will have good ideas about which genetic condition may be related to a nerve receptor, and there should be scope for people to follow trails of potentially useful discoveries – but if we are expecting patients to take part in trials and also, as taxpayers and charity fundraisers, pay for it all surely the community should be asked, what is most important to know? As the Alltrials campaign has shown (see Chapter 4), much research is simply never published – an easy way to skew results into looking better than they in reality are – but the research may not be asking the questions that patients want the answers to.

The James Lind Alliance, set up in 2004, has been instrumental in addressing these questions.[51] The alliance brings researchers and patients together to work out their shared priorities for research. Patients are no longer being told to follow doctor's orders but are instead treated as collaborative colleagues. Not only is this ethical, but it is also more efficient and less wasteful, because this process ensures that the agreed-upon research will be useful. This is a profound change and it has been achieved through the most fundamental of human devices at the disposal of the NHS: conversations between people.

The biggest and best resource the NHS has are the people who work in it and use it. The NHS in Hampshire asked patients with mental illness what kind of support they needed. It found that unwanted attendances at A&E decreased when they set up a drop-in cafe which hosted psychiatric staff.[52] It's logical, simple: you won't find gaps in healthcare unless you talk to the people who know where they are. Patients and families can help to spot mistakes in healthcare when staff do not, thus enabling systems to improve faster and better.[53] A review of evidence revealed research about why people didn't attend hospital appointments for diabetes care, but very little of it asking the invitees themselves. When they were asked, young people with type 1 diabetes explained that they were keen to attend but afraid that they would be scolded for having '*poor control'* – an insight that professionals need to know (because frightening people into attending is therefore far less likely to be helpful than offering understanding and support).[54]

This doesn't happen enough. There are numerous top-down assumptions made by healthcare systems which have not asked first. For example, as mentioned in Chapter 4, the National Institute for Health and Care Excellence (NICE) has written guidance for statin-prescribing when people are calculated as having a 10% risk of cardiovascular disease in the following ten years. The committee has said: *'For some interventions, the Guideline Development Group is confident that, given the information it has looked at, most patients would choose the intervention.'* [55] But when people are asked what kind of benefit they would want for the commitment to take a regular statin, the answers are highly variable. One-third of people are willing to take statins even if they only gain a month of extra life, but 15% of people are willing to take the medication only if there are two or more years of life to be gained and 10% would only take the tablets if more than ten years of life could be gained. Yet 99% of people would have have no, or less than two years, of additional lifespan because of the tablet. We should not assume that because some doctors decree a long-term treatment worthwhile, so will everyone else.[56]

Exactly the same finding has been made when people are invited to take part in choosing their care. In medicine there are often grey areas. You can have a different operation with a higher success rate but a longer recovery period; or medication that doesn't work as well and has some unpredictable side effects, but for which there is no need for a hospital stay. Calling this *'what are my options'* conversation *'shared decision-making'* is relatively new and only started to be seriously researched in the late 1990s.[57] Sharing decisions about using antibiotics in general practice can reduce their use,[58] which is important given that antibiotic resistance is a troubling consequence of prescribing them.[59] Formalised *'decision aids'* (which can be online or paper based) clearly brings people closer to making the decisions they value.[60] These aids also reduce elective surgery and patients are just as satisfied afterwards – it results in less and better medicine.[61] It's important not to overreach what the evidence says about the power of shared decision-making to reduce costs,[62] but of fundamental importance is the fact that patients are a heterogenous group with both autonomy and legitimate views on which medicine is, and is not, worth taking.

This is seen most clearly at the end of life. Some doctors have described too much medicine in older people as *attempts at curative but futile and unwanted but difficult-to-resist care* as *elder abuse* [63] because it removes people from their own homes and subjects them to unpleasant or harmful treatments that have no realistic prospect of success. More broadly, when death is near, it's clear that doctors often recommend more treatment for patients than they would wish for themselves.[64] This is especially troubling because most people say they want to die at home, but more intensive treatment in hospitals results in more people dying somewhere apart from it.

It's clear to me that healthcare works best when patients and doctors are plainly on the same side. When financial motivations are kept to a minimum. When the values of continuity of care and ongoing relationships are cherished. When patients are encouraged and facilitated to direct research goals and to participate as equals. When people who use services are enabled to shape how they are delivered. When patients are properly listened to, given *clean* advice about benefit and risk, and enabled to make choices of high value to each. When vocationally motivated doctors publish as much data as they have on what they are doing, but do not overreach conclusions, are not punished for it, and think critically of what they are doing, who they are doing it for and why.

Is this so impossible? We already have many of the necessary ingredients. But we need several more things: a moral purpose that is shared with the society that funds the NHS; and a commitment to ensure that the collective resources are used with care, wisdom and evidence.

Interview

John D. Townsend, NHS patient

I've just had to give up, after having two bouts of chemotherapy. Both times put me in hospital with a chest infection. The oncologist said any more would kill me, so I'm not having the rest. It's just the way things are.

Three years ago I had just come back from holiday. But within a few weeks I had lost an awful lot of weight, and my appetite had gone. I knew that wasn't right, and it prompted me to go to the doctor's. I went to my GP. She examined me, and rather than blurting it out and coming out with the word 'cancer' – she didn't know if I would get upset or not – we sat in her office and she said 'What do you think it is?' I looked her in the eye and said, 'I think it's bowel cancer'. She seemed taken aback and said 'well, it might not be', but she would get me referred over to the hospital. And within a few days I had a thick package from the hospital about all the tests I'd to have.

It was very efficient. She treated me very well. She listens to what I have to say – and she must have other patients, some that are never satisfied, some that are bloody awkward; but I knew her already. It's got to the point where if I meet her in the street, she not only knows that I'm one of her patients, but will wave across the marketplace, and call me by my first name. It's that sort of relationship. It makes a difference.

I've been lucky. I've had doctors and nurses who listen to what patients say, and don't have an arrogant attitude. It means they get to hear what is important. I've felt taken seriously. I'd never had a day off work through sickness in 27 years till this happened. I now don't have any plans at all. I enjoy seeing my grandchildren but I am so tired now, I just want to sit and close my eyes. A year ago they told me I had months to live, and that I wasn't strong enough for chemo. But I did get stronger, and that's when they gave me the chemo. But I can't get any more of that – the oncologist thinks it would finish me off.

So I'm biding my time. I'm planning to stay at home, with my wife there, but I don't mind going into the hospice. I go there once a week already. I enjoy my grandchildren, but I can't do much else. I have confidence that I will be looked after and that the district nurses and my doctor will see me – I don't need them right now.

You only ever hear bad things about the NHS. I've said to my wife before – I don't know where all these bloody complaints come from. Where are these people? You never get to hear about the good things.

9

Keeping the NHS Alive

The banks were too important to fail. The NHS is being allowed to. How can we ensure it still exists, free at the point of use, for our children and theirs?

We need our NHS to run on evidence, moral value and humanity. We need to ask for the right evidence, put evidence before policy, make no policy without cognisance of the evidence, and always consider the harms.

The NHS is profoundly affected by policymaking – whether health checks, dementia screening, the decision to implement the Health and Social Care Act, the effects of social care cuts, or food or alcohol law. Policymaking in healthcare takes place frequently at all levels – from a practice policy to follow-up raised cholesterol tests to deciding nationally how to organise and run vaccination programmes. Some of these policies are made by health professionals and patients alone, with little or no input from political policymakers. Other health policies are proposed by politicians (like the sugar tax, or minimum alcohol price) and are then consulted on, with academics invited to discuss and debate the issues. But some other policies are set while overriding the built-in safety catches of the other types, designed to ensure that evidence is followed and harm is minimised.

In the second type, academics may already have offered or lobbied their views to government. Academics independently create and publish evidence, and it is usually later synthesised into more reliable reviews of evidence. But this is a slow and often tedious[1] process when government needs rapid, clear scientific appraisal, where the facts and uncertainties are made clear. Systematic reviews can be slow and may not answer the needs of policymakers. Even though *good policymakers will always be asking the question, "what is the opportunity cost of this new initiative?"*,[2] the reality is that opportunity costs are seldom appreciated. The priorities of politicians may be dramatically different from those of patients and clinicians. Chris Whitty, an epidemiologist and previously Chief Scientific Adviser at the UK Department for International Development, writes: '*An 80% right paper before a policy decision is made is worth ten 95% right papers afterwards.*' Academics, who are often paid in part or full by the state, could do more to become fundamentally involved with not just challenging and appraising proposed policy but also explaining what evidence-based policy would look like.[3]

Paul Cairney, professor of politics and public policy, argues that academics should deliver their work in ways that are useful to policymakers – who may not be politically able to use '*the evidence*' as it is usually created: instead academics wanting to have impact need to bend to the political machine '*to engage in a normative enterprise that can increase impact at the expense of objectivity*'. Yet this would not be enough to ensure that health policymaking stopped avoidable harms and would not create the system change we need: the way we make policy in healthcare needs to be rationalised and made safer.

There are now multiple, educated agencies in the UK offering to try and make policymaking more evidence-based and cognisant of the history of similar issues. The Alliance for Useful Evidence, together with the Institute for Government and Sense about Science have created an '*evidence transparency tool*', which allows government departments to be '*rated*' in terms of how they use evidence to create policy.[4] History and Policy, a non-partisan network of academic historians, offers historical research in order for contemporary policymakers to '*avoid reinventing the wheel and repeating past mistakes*'.[5] In the US there are organisations like the Center for Evidence-based Policy and the Coalition for Evidence-Based Policy (now the Laura and John Arnold Foundation).[6] In Australia, the Grattan Institute.[7] The need to generate evidence is not unique to medicine (see the Campbell Collaboration for a library of reviews of evidence in social policy)[8] and evidence-based policymaking is not and should not be solely relevant to medicine.[9] However, we have a major problem when secretaries of state for health declare, *'We must only support effective interventions that deliver proven benefits,'* [10] but then propose things that are either inadequately tested or are shown not to work. If we don't put money where it has the best chance of serving patients, we flush it away in the process, as well as the time, effort and energy of staff, patients and administrators. We simply don't have the money or human lives to waste.

It is clear that there are many committed and enormously able individuals working in and outside of government who want to ensure the stability and endurance of the NHS. But the systematic way in which policy decisions are made leaves the NHS wide open to that policy being based on poor or no evidence.

Here are nine proposals for making better health policy.

1. Put an effective buffer between government and the NHS on policymaking
Despite the efforts to put evidence-based decision-making into Whitehall,[11] the fact is that multiple non-evidence-based policies (like the increasing tick boxes of the GP contract, or many targets in hospital care) have become policies with multi-million pound spending sprees, bypassing the checks and balances (NICE and UKNSC) that were meant to offer evidence-based advice (not to proceed).

From the Health and Social Care Act, to Healthchecks, dementia screening, the now jettisoned care.data project, Private Finance Initiatives, Independent Sector Treatment Centres, management consultancies, NHS homeopathic hospitals, GP doors opening to empty waiting rooms on Sundays, the private sector transferring work to the NHS, the now-closed Strategic Business Team,[12] companies offering 'culture change' which costs £5 million rather than under

300,000,[13] still a vast amount, ludicrous payouts to chief executives: every single new policy needs interrogated by asking, is this cost-effective, evidence-based, and beneficial to patients and staff? And if so, what must we stop spending money or time on in order to fit this in? All this money that could have been spent on evidence-based interventions like safe staffing levels.

These policy failures override safety catches in pursuit of political dogma. NICE has been the best example of evidence-based policymaking in practice in recent times, for it has been devolved to make difficult decisions on funding using the best available evidence. It has, though, been undermined by two things. The first is too many ties to industry, creating conflicts of interest, as will be discussed below, and the second is being undermined by political activity.

The Cancer Drugs Fund is a case in point. It was created by government to subvert the political problem of highly expensive drugs being requested by (often terminally ill) patients when the funding had not been agreed by NICE. There was huge media hostility towards a Department of Health, depicted as being uncaring, apparently willing to let people die rather than fund their drug. Far from being rarely used when NICE were too slow to appraise a promising treatment, it ended up funding one in five people starting chemotherapy. Yet half the drugs being prescribed through the Cancer Drugs Fund had already been judged by NICE as not cost-effective. The costs increased from £38 million to £416 million over four years, before the National Audit Office described it as *'not sustainable'* and lacking information about whether it was effective. The Cancer Drugs Fund was essentially a back door to subvert the decision-making process that NICE was using and only available to people with cancer, and not for other conditions.[14]

In many ways, NICE protects government from having to make unpopular but fair decisions. It has a clear process of involving patients and of creating draft guidance, which is then shared for discussion. But it appears that when an idea is politically advantageous, policy is squeezed through even when there is a clear method of independent appraisal and evidence already exists to show that it either does not work or is harmful. Further, it creates a fig-leaf of an excuse that something useful is being done, when it is not.

This is not sustainable – and it is wasteful. Indeed, as healthcare improvement researchers have stated: *'It is difficult to escape the impression that primary care policy is being influenced more by an unhealthy combination of ideology and political pragmatism, than by the research evidence of what works.'*[15] There needs to be clear buffers between non-evidenced political policy and patients in the NHS. David Halpern, director of the previously governmental and now private Behavioural Insights Unit (commonly known as the *'Nudge Unit'*), has written from Whitehall:

'There will always be many factors that go into a policy decision, such as the legitimate political concerns of government. But the wise and appropriate use of evidence should be at the heart of policy too: what are the problems, what are its causes, and what might work to change it?' [16]

But we have a system where experts submit evidence to parliament showing that the imposed contract on junior doctors[17] is not mathematically feasible, may breach duty of care to employees' health and risk higher levels of fatigue, which would directly impact on patient safety:[18] but can be absolutely ignored. The evidence went in a month before a health minister said plainly, of the junior doctors' contract: *'...we have to move ahead with implementation. That train has now left the station.'*[19] Unpublished academic work was used to support both the Health and Social Care Act and the change to junior doctors contracts: on publication, both conclusions were vigorously contested in the academic community.[20] This is not evidence-based policymaking. It is party political cherry picking.

A mature political system should be able to put party political differences aside and look to co-operation and shared priorities. Bevan, in 1945, said as much of doctors: *'I know very well I am not going to succeed in my task by bullying methods. I have to meet them across the table and try to break down their suspicions,'* he explained. *'Therefore I hope they will not come and meet me as if I were an antagonist on the other side of the table; on the contrary, I am one whose enthusiasm for democratic medicine is as great as their own.'* [21] Indeed, that is what Heidi Alexander, then Labour shadow health secretary, had in mind when she, along with colleagues in the Liberal Democrat, Scottish Nationalist and Conservative parties, wrote to Jeremy Hunt to suggest cross-party working.[22] They proposed to Hunt that better evidence should be sought and a new contract piloted. This was rejected as *'opportunism'.*[23] Certainly, a democratically elected government should be free to campaign on a platform for change. But that change could be ineffective and harmful if it is not based on careful examination of the evidence. The ethos of NICE needs to be strengthened, made more focused and even more transparent, able to wed academia and policymaking in real time.

This recurrent problem needs a better solution. We already have the ideology of the NHS, whose founding principles (see page 7) arose from a broad political consensus. What we do not have is a clear strategy about how to use evidence to enact those principles in policymaking.

We already have nationally funded institutions like NICE in England and the Scottish Medicines Consortium, which do the job of appraising evidence and making cost-effectiveness judgements. Exactly the same could happen for politicians who have policy ideas: tell the evidence agencies about the problem that you are trying to solve and they can tell you what is known, what is not known and what needs to be tested. Had this been done for dementia screening, it would never have been rolled out. Money would have been saved. General practitioners would have been able to pay more attention to their patients' concerns. Patients would not have written to newspapers in despair at their consultation being hijacked. And we would have realised that the true numbers of people with dementia were less than first thought, and been glad that we hadn't wasted all that effort needlessly. Similarly, had Alexander's ideas for gathering and testing evidence been formalised, doctors' strikes and ill will could have been averted.

The NHS needs long-term stability and an inbuilt mechanism that protects it from poor policy. It is time to disentangle it from short-term party politics and entrust it to longer term, cross-bench, collaborative oversight, where evidence-based policymaking is married to the founding principles of the NHS.

2. Publicly and permanently declare potential conflicts of interest, but insist on minimising them

Our major political parties say the same: they want to cherish the NHS. Using the NHS for short-term political gain should become unacceptable. The ascent of a political career should not come at the expense of the NHS. Nor should a political career lead to the private or management consultancy health sector after retirement.

Medical careers can also corrupt what is in the best interests of the NHS. The worst example is probably that of a consultant who will see a patient privately and then place them on the NHS waiting list for further treatment, meaning that they are seen before others who have not yet had their first NHS appointment. This should be possible to fix. There is a good argument for sealing the private sector off from the NHS entirely and not allowing hospital doctors to work for both: further, the private medicine sector provides little training for junior doctors and seldom takes part in clinical research. Yet it takes delivery of state-trained doctors and has been accused of transferring care to NHS services when people are no longer profitable to the private sector. Doctors who straddle both sectors are in an invidious position. The growth of nitpicking in the 2004 GP contract has created constant conflicts for doctors, who have been lured into a money-earning, tick-box system, which have effectively hijacked the consultation away from what the patient wants to talk about. GPs need to operate more like consultants, who are paid per unit of time, publish their data, and try and understand and improve on it. The status of GPs as independent contractors to the NHS has probably resulted in NHS stability and cost savings until recent times, but we are in a different era now. Under the HSCA, general practice is ripe for takeover from the private sector. I suspect there is no universal solution, but GPs who want to change from being independent contractors working to the contract to a more professional, fairly contracted model – that of being directly employed by the NHS – should be enabled to do so.

Financial conflicts are only just being dragged into the open. We know that almost £40 million a year is paid to healthcare professionals in the UK: but we do not know all the details of to whom and for what.[24] This is immensely troubling, especially given that some doctors – including those responsible for writing guidelines for other doctors on prescribing – take money from numerous pharmaceuticals (to the extent that some describe themselves as *promiscuous* with the number of drug companies they choose to accept fees from).[25] The Association of British Pharmaceutical Industries (ABPI) has agreed to publish prospective payments from 2015 (in 2016). However, this will only be with the consent of the healthcare professional. This is needless: the ABPI could have made the agreement to disclosure into a condition of employment and it could be permanently published at point of contract. There is an urgent need for this. It remains to be seen how effective a voluntary register will be (meantime, a test-of-concept website, whopaysthisdoctor.org, which I had a hand in organising, exists to allow doctors with and without financial conflicts to make a voluntary entry).

Commissioning has given professionals a disgraceful opportunity to market themselves to *pharma*. Pharmacists and managers have been alleged to have simultaneously acted as consultants to *pharma* to get drugs of their choice onto the recommended lists used by GPs.[26]

In 2016, NHS England decided it would strengthen the management of conflicts of interest[27] – but without an emphasis on the need to avoid them, staff could still do '*dual working*' (as a pharmacist or doctor some days, but as director of a consultancy on other days). There are also counter-currents where the Department of Trade and Industry encourages clinical commissioning groups (CCGs) to make use of pharmacists, employed via pharmaceutical companies to access people's medical records and make recommendations of new treatments.[28] However, this is currently being treated not as a '*conflict*' but an '*innovation*'.

The General Medical Council is paid hundreds of pounds by doctors annually to keep a register of their professional status. It would be straightforward to ask doctors to annually submit a register of declared interests, which would be published and could be searched by anyone and everyone. To make this statutory would require an Act of parliament. In the meantime, it could be done on a trial basis and should be extended to pharmacists, nurses and hospital managers.

Declaring interests, however, is not enough. While some conflicts cannot be avoided (my deep love for the NHS may create a bias), others can. So it should not be permissible for doctors to accept '*pharma*' money for consultancy if they are also giving advice to guideline committees on what drugs to use. I don't think it is safe to receive postgraduate education from '*pharma*' either: there is clear evidence that doctors who receive payments from '*pharma*' prescribe drugs differently (that is, in favour of more expensive brand names) than doctors who do not.[29] This is no surprise. '*Pharma*' has known this, through access to doctor-level prescribing data, for years. They would not waste money on marketing that did not work.

NICE and its Scottish equivalent, the Scottish Intercollegiate Guidelines Network (SIGN), have had to contend with similar problems. Accusations of bias in guideline writing have festered for years. NICE says that it is not conflicted (despite having employed people who later absented themselves because of a conflict).[30] When the Department for Trade and Industry allows lightly checked '*pharma*' access into the NHS it calls it '*innovation*'.[31] While chairs of NICE committees are not allowed to have personal or non-personal financial ties to commercial organisations, committee members themselves are. 'Personal financial non-specific' monies have to be declared, but beyond that, professionals who also act as consultants or directors to the pharmaceutical industry can take a full part in committees. This is surely insufficient; if professionals choose to take up positions which create financial conflicts of interest, committees should choose members without them.

3. We need to talk about money

The NHS is given lots of money, but not enough. In terms of percentage of GDP, we spend less than France, Portugal or Greece.[32] If we want more front line staff, we have to pay for them. But we also waste money– not just in evidence-free ideological jollies like the Health and Social Care Act, but as in 1. and 2. above. As I write, most NHS Trusts are heading for 'unprecedented deficits', projected to be £2.3 billion in 2016. The normally conservative King's Fund asked if the NHS was in a 'financial crisis'.[33] The government's spending review of 2015 announced that NHS England would receive £10 billion more a year in real terms by 2020/21 than in 2014/15. In fact, this was found by the Health Committee to be £4.5 billion in real terms.[34] This has been much less than expected and does not take account of the fact that £22 billion worth of NHS 'efficiency savings' were announced in 2014, to be met by the end of the parliamentary term ending in 2020.[35] Simultaneously, public spending as a whole is being cut by £600 million, on top of the £200 million already sheared; the real effect is being felt in council staff redundancies. Since social care and healthcare are two sides of the same coin, it is difficult to see how this can be done safely. In 2016, the Public Accounts Committee expressed 'our concerns that the overly ambitious efficiency target had damaged Trusts' financial positions'.[36]

Monitor had told Foundation Trusts to fill vacancies 'only where essential' because they faced 'unprecedented financial challenge'.[37] Given that the Francis inquiry found that low staffing levels caused harm, Monitor's instruction risks repeating history. Nevertheless, Trusts have been warned that if they fail to *'balance the books without compromising patient care'* their governing boards will be suspended.[38] As a joint report from the King's Fund, Nuffield Trust and The Health Foundation put it: *'In the face of unprecedented financial pressures and rising demand for services, this is not sustainable.'*[39]

Astonishingly, in 2016 the Department of Health has proceeded with changes to accountancy practices, which include reclassifying assets in ways which an analyst from the Nuffield Trust said entered *'the area of fiddles'*.[40]

General practice is in an ongoing crisis, with experienced doctors retiring early and practices being kept afloat by locums: 20% of GP practices in London are considering closing their doors.[41]

Yet right in the middle of these cuts, acutely in the centre of this squeeze, the government went to war with junior doctors over their contract under the promise of a *'7-day NHS'*. Even if the policy did even the mortality rates across the week (and that is not proven to be the case), the increased costs it entails means that it is prohibitively expensive.[42] How can it be possible to leave staff posts vacant to balance the books, while at the same time increasing the services on offer? It makes no sense. The UK spends less on funding the NHS than many other northern European countries like Norway and Sweden, and far less than Denmark, France and Germany.[43] Another term for deficits would be *'gaps caused by underfunding'*. The British Social Attitudes Survey of 2015 found that 92% of people believe the NHS is facing a funding problem, but most did not want to spend any more tax on it.[44] If we can't have five star funding, we can't have a five star service.

We can't have it both ways. Either corners are cut to save money, which means lower quality, riskier care, or more money will be needed. In the meantime, money that is spent on non-evidence-based care risks being wasted entirely.

The NHS was launched with the intention of meeting people's needs regardless of their ability to pay. This has been undermined by the uprising of multiple, easy-access web applications and internet services offering private GP services. These companies market themselves as offering instant access to GPs, and advertise themselves to NHS GPs as a way of making easier money with less stress. Patients pay up front and generally have longer appointments – though some companies expressly exclude treating mental illness or chronic conditions. The contract GPs hold with the NHS means that they cannot see their own patients privately. These companies will be responsible for the absurd situation where someone without money may wait weeks for an NHS appointment at surgery A. If they are able to pay, though, they could get a quick appointment at a GP surgery B down the road from their own, while patients from the nearby surgery B could equally pay to have faster access to surgery A. But only if you have money. Drawing staff into the private sector from the NHS will seal its destruction. And of course, the private sector does not pay for the training of doctors in the first place. The covenant between the NHS, medicine and society is being thus corrupted. GPs being salaried would protect the NHS: but only if the contract was fair and trusted enough.

4. Professionalism is a better motivator than fear

Just as patients have been treated only as passive recipients of healthcare, most healthcare practitioners have been treated as only passive re-enactors of policy handed down from above. The atmosphere that many staff members work in is one of fear (charges of manslaughter, bullying, the consequences of missed targets), stress (staff shortages, physical and mental fatigue, working beyond contracted hours), humiliation (publication of CQC scores, threats to give traffic light ratings to GPs, little right of reply to degrading negative public feedback) and frustration (a feeling that management thinks a job is never being done well, or finished). This is occurring across the NHS, both in staff that are more visible to patients[45] and those less so.[46]

The result is a mixture of burnout, early retirement and resentment. When complaints from patients and families

– justified or not – are added, the staff that were already giving extra hours, ideas and integrity start to dissolve under the pressure. The consequences are staff shortages and even poorer care for patients. The management 'cure' is to apply more pressure to reach more targets. It's easy to see how a stressed system simply degrades.

Part of the answer has to be to treat people fundamentally better. Work should be enjoyable, usually pleasant and fulfilling. It is impossible for staff who are bullied and threatened to be open and fearless about reporting mistakes, errors, near misses and definitive harm. It is impossible for a place that is half-staffed to do as good a job as a properly staffed facility would. Complaints processes should take place in a 'just culture' – we need to accept that perfection is impossible, well-intentioned human mistakes will happen, and good-enough medicine requires enough on-the-ground resources that we will have to pay for.

Instead of staff being seen as a bunch of disparate people to be managed into submission, it would be far better to appeal to human values. People who enter the healthcare professions are interviewed and expected to describe their vocation. They are usually satisfied by doing a good job. They tend to have their morale better protected when they work in tight teams. They will often work overtime for free and fill gaps, and this good nature should be appreciated and cherished, not exploited. See, for example, the lauded Netherlands' model of district nursing where small teams, able to make rapid decisions with minimal bureaucracy, look after patients' entire social care and healthcare needs, which saves on cost while improving quality.[47] Staff who are treated well themselves will treat patients and families better.

5. Patients and families can help to get things right
I would not suggest that patients and families should take on responsibility for their care when they are too ill to do so or don't want to. Yet people generally have to go on dealing with conditions and all the burdens associated with them

well beyond their limited and, in the community, occasional contact with healthcare staff. As one patient – who also happened to be a doctor – described the situation:

'*In my first rotation … I lost track within the first week of how many outpatient appointments I sat in on. I didn't really think anything of them—they are just another 15-minute slot of time filled with learning in a very busy day. As a patient, my perspective couldn't be more different. I have one appointment with my consultant a year, and spend weeks planning and preparing, then a month recovering emotionally.*' [48]

The modern terms are '*self-management*' and '*activated patients*', researching their own condition, making proactive choices, and discussing or feeding in to broader groups, or patients who are more engaged with monitoring and tracking their own conditions. But I don't think this describes it quite well enough: '*self-management*' is what everyone does for themselves most of the time, and is nothing out of the ordinary. As I have described (see page 204), the time has come to move on from professionals '*doing things*' to patients. We have to work together, using the moral principles of the NHS in tandem with evidence-based medicine to guide us. This can be as straightforward as considering what are the best ways to write appointment letters to patients.[49]

I think Alison Cameron (the first '*patient*' to graduate from the NHS Leadership Academy has it right:

'[this is] *not about professionals having to relinquish power in an already chaotic and uncertain climate, but about strengthening the power base so there is more of it to go around. Patient leaders are often not in the hierarchy, so we have more freedom to look outwards rather than upwards. This makes us potentially powerful allies for professionals who are struggling to challenge the status quo.*'[50]

If healthcare professionals are fed up with the political focus on things that don't matter, it is doubly effective to tackle what is '*coming down from above*', together. Far from being each other's enemy, the natural position should be alongside each other. Yet the system we work in serially dismisses or diminishes the importance and need for individual patient views.[51] Much of healthcare is about human relationships and being: talking, thinking, choosing, waiting, living with uncertainty. Often there are no right 'answers' but just less wrong ones, or decisions that are easier to live with. It is, instead, our relationships with patients and colleagues which define our work.[52]

6. Publish transparent data: not 'intelligent', but wise
We are producing mountains of data. We have data on who attended, when, what was prescribed, who was referred, what tests were done, how often prescriptions were collected, how many times I clicked a box ...

Some of this information is very useful. Some of it causes more problems than it could ever have solved. Take the case of Bristol University Health Service, which was castigated by the CQC about the shingles vaccine. The CQC's data would have shown that no one had received it. Yet it is only available to certain groups of older people aged 70 and above.[53] The practice has no one registered with it in this age group because its services are available only to students.[54] A little bit of common sense was all that was needed. Similarly, the claim made in parliament that '*across all key specialties, in only 10% of our hospitals are patients seen by a consultant within 14 hours of being admitted at the weekend*' is plainly false to anyone who has ever worked in hospitals at the weekend. It fails the test of common sense, never mind wisdom. Indeed, when the same data was analysed by the statistician David Speigelhalter, he diagnosed the statement as having '*two errors and one misleading claim*' because the average amount of patients seen by a consultant within 14 hours was 79%.[55]

Statistics are often used, as the poet Andrew Lang said, as a drunk man uses a lamppost – for support, not illumination.[56] I would go further; too often statistics are used to create fear and humiliate rather than achieve understanding and improvement. Just as medicine historically has been slow to appreciate uncertainty and the importance of '*unknown unknowns'*, we are keen to use a tsunami of data to draw conclusions that may not be safe nor accurate.

This is not an argument against transparency, which I support (de-identified to protect patient privacy: for example, in publication of prescription data or mortality rates). Just as important, though, is twinning data with a clear appreciation of the uncertainties and hazards it contains.[57] Often it is not clear what the data represents – for example, a surgeon with high mortality rates may be the best surgeon there is, taking on the most difficult, high-risk patients whom other surgeons turn down, and who would certainly die without surgery. Big data sets should be used to ask better questions, but they can only rarely fully answer them. When problems are found, they should be identified and dealt with under the principle that everyone should be kept as safe as possible. This means patients and families, of course, but it also means staff, who are at risk themselves of burnout and distress as a result of working in poor conditions. The way to do this, of course, is to work with staff and patients, not against them.

7. Legislation and guidelines for safety, efficiency and long-term relationships

The HSCA in England has created a marketplace that is not rooted in either an appreciation of the evidence or interest in it. This creates an ongoing diversion of money and time into following the legal processes for commissioning. The HSCA could be repealed. Recent attempts to do so via the NHS Reinstatement Bill, which was supported from the front by Caroline Lucas of the Greens with cross-party support,[58] was talked out of its second reading by filibustering.[59] The campaign on this continues. The HSCA was meant to lower costs and raise quality, but we now have evidence that the new private companies providing NHS general practice services are either performing worse or no better than traditional services.[60]

Repealing the HSCA would be a very clear way to ensure that the NHS was more efficient, saving money by stopping commissioning and tendering processes that don't add to patient care. An estimated £4.5 billion is spent on maintaining the NHS market.[61] This wipes out any increase in funding. It seems that the ideology of party politics is a hindrance to evidence-based, high-quality healthcare.

NICE has the power to mandate the availability of drugs or treatments it has recommended,[62] which ensures that everyone has the right of access to the beneficial treatments no matter where they live. However, the ideal of ending postcode lotteries has been eroded as cuts to services and local commissioning decisions have caused differences in the provision of things such as fertility treatment.[63] NICE had been generating evidence reviews into safe-staffing, publishing guidance in 2014 that one nurse should look after no more than eight patients on adult wards at a time.[64] However, this was not made into a legal requirement. After two years of work, in 2015 the Department of Health told NICE to stop its research into recommendations for safe-staffing levels.[65] NICE did eventually publish the remainder in 2016.[66] Managers however wrote to Trusts saying that the 1:8 staffing ratio was *a guide not a requirement*,[67] which, given that staffing was a crucial problem in Mid Staffs and getting it better was a totem of the Francis Report, would seem very risky indeed. Indeed, despite the research on nurse numbers and safety, 42% of nurses surveyed by Unison were responsible, on a spot check, for more than eight patients.[68] Evidence from Australia and the US east coast shows mandated nurse staffing levels – which vary with the type of ward and patients – are possible and that they result in higher quality care and lower stress for staff.[69] The CQC would neither recommend safe staffing levels or mandate them.[70] The chief regulator of NHS Improvement told NHS Trusts that higher staffing levels was unaffordable: *'we'll be saying we can't afford it, that's not something that justified, there's no evidence for it, it's not delivering better outcomes'* – despite of all the evidence to the contrary.[71] Some *'efficiencies'* are simply harmful.

We need to mandate the things that matter. Poor staff

numbers are associated with an increased risk of death. Building inefficiencies into the NHS – such as the legal processes of the HSCA – misuses resources and wastes money. Hospitals have been repeatedly warned not to spend on staffing in order to make budgets[72] – exactly the kind of target Francis told us was so dangerous.

Understaffing is likely to get worse without massive and rapid effort: Brexit may make international recruitment more difficult, and the Migration Advisory Committee has warned of the lack of adequate long term planning and impact of cost-savings on ensuring enough nurses to staff the NHS.[73] Vacancies get propped up with locum and agency staff, more expensive and less stable – a medical staffing market in action. The NHS is reliant on it's people: but at every crisis, this keeps being seen as a bit of a surprise.

8. Unseen services are vital services; not everything that matters can be counted

I write as a GP and this book will have weaknesses and strengths because of that. However, most healthcare does take place in the community over long periods of time. As Iona Heath's family doctor told her when she told him she was going to do medicine: *'In general practice the people stay and the diseases come and go. In hospital the diseases stay and the people come and go.'* [74] Primary care – across general practice, physiotherapy, social care and pharmacy – is the network that protects secondary care from inefficiency by selecting which patients needs their services.[75] Primary and secondary care services depend on each other to work well.

This is increasingly impossible. Unmet social care needs simply end up either causing harm to the person and their family or ends up being dealt with less efficiently and humanely in the NHS. People will be admitted to hospital when they could have stayed at home if they had had better support (whether in terms of accommodation, home nursing visits or being unable to cook for themselves), and they will stay longer in hospital beds if they cannot be discharged to a safe place.

Community care suffers from a lack of glamour. The carers who give bed baths and dispose of the urine and faeces of people dying at home are likely to be either family, friends or the lowest-paid staff in the NHS. The district nurses who criss-cross over the community patch to deliver medicines, dressings, deathcare and solace with dwindling staff do huge amounts to contain needs at home. Like most things that work, it's only when it goes wrong that we notice and get involved. But no one can sustainably provide as good care when more is asked of fewer staff.

Similarly, mental healthcare, mainly submerged deep in the community and usually kept far from the bright hospital lights, does long-term, relationship-based work that is often invisible despite its profound value. Mental illness is often less visible, for shame and stigma still haunt disclosure. One-third of community services are now run by non-NHS providers,[76] which means that it can be harder to keep tabs on who is doing what and how. The laboratory staff, porters and hospital cleaners are often barely visible to the outside world but the NHS system crumbles without them to underpin the services.

9. Professional, human values at all times

Working as a GP in the NHS is the best job in the world. On my worst days, getting good care for patients seems like running somewhere between an assault and an obstacle course, with tedious computer entries and pointless paperwork. I feel powerless to run less late, and am overwhelmed with sadness for a family as they prepare to part with a mother, father or child, or the need to tell someone else that a test result means bad news, or am frustrated with the difficulty of trying to organise an overnight carer for a dying patient.

But then there are the days where I am able to ignore most of the obstructive bureaucracy, concentrate more on what people say, talk about what people and families want to do, and reach that moment when I finally understand what it is that someone is worried about, or where I am the first person who is told about domestic violence or rape, or realise that a patient is likely to die soon, and offer to start a conversation about the future which is likely to unfold over the weeks ahead. These are days when I can talk to my colleagues about whether I am doing the right thing, or when the nurses come along to tell me how patients are doing, and it is the kind of day when, on my way home, I bump into someone whose depression I was involved in treating a decade ago, and she greets me and tells me that she is doing very, very well.

Values have to be first – before evidence, before policy, before politics. The joy in medicine is still there to be had. It rests on relationships. When we make the systems we work in better, we can ourselves work better. There is no better work. This has been recognised for generations, and was in evidence at the very beginning of the NHS.

The NHS is the best practical demonstration of human values that exists. But it is not a creature run on magic. The human values the NHS is founded on have been eroded in the endless squabbling over which political philosophy gets a shot next. Endless disruption, conflicted interests and failing to pay attention to what works and what we need have caused repeated, avoidable harm.

We can choose to cherish the NHS, but to do so will also mean abandoning the interference from party politics. Instead, a cross-party collaboration is required, founded on marrying the humanity and moral agency of the NHS with high-quality, evidence-based policymaking. It can be done; the tools are at our disposal. The question is whether we can be decent and insightful enough to realise that to ensure that the NHS remains our shared heritage, and to keep creating it out of humans for the generations ahead, we must throw off the shackles of party political ownership.

Epilogue

As I finished writing and started the editing process for this book, the next upheaval emerged. STPs – Sustainability and Transformation Plans. These are the iteration of the Five Year Forward View, the NHS England publication which promises more money to general practice. But there is no point spending more money on general practice if it's wasted on things that don't work. This is even more critical when the NHS is being starved of resources; we can't afford to make mistakes. The NHS is calling these STPs 'collective discussion forums'. GPs have said they have been excluded from discussions. Some have already started talking about cutting hospital bed numbers, and Pulse, a medical newspaper, asked all STPs to share their plans in August 2016, and all refused. In Scotland, 'cluster working' has been launched, GPs working in groups to organise and plan services. In common is the idea that general practice should be done 'at scale' – what isn't feasible to be done in small numbers becomes rational at larger. Some of this might be good: for example, additional services could be organised at greater convenience for a large number of patients near where they live. But in a climate of austerity, the message that keeps coming through is instead of cost savings to scale. Some areas are proposing merging or closing GP practices, decreasing the number of appointments available with doctors, and using technology-enabled care instead. Yet the evidence for this being safe or effective is lacking. The re-dis-organisation is trying to do more with less, and there does come a point at which cost-effective efficiency savings can no longer be made – at least, savings on the things that we are being given a choice about.

We need new choices. We need to be allowed at least the option of paying for the NHS we need. We also need the option of rejecting short term political policy making in favour of making mature cross party decisions drawing on evidence and expertise, freeing the NHS from the legacy of damaged through the shorter-term need for political parties to claim successes for themselves or blame failures on others.

I love what the NHS stands for. If we want it always to stand, free at the point of use, we need a serious national conversation, with facts, not fancy, and citizens who are prepared to engage with evidence and uncertainty while remembering that the NHS should be there for every one of us according to need. The NHS should be the best of us, for all of us.

September 2016

Thanks

To the people who agreed to make the time to be interviewed for this book: thank you for illuminating dark corners and explaining the evolution, nature and problems of the NHS so well.

I read a great many books and papers to help me write this one, and Iain Chalmers, Julian Tudor Hart, Iona Heath, Trish Greenhalgh, David Owen and Mary Dixon-Woods' work has been especially useful.

Martin Wagner and Maria Pinter have continued to support me with their usual generous kindness. Thank you to Christopher Westhorp for editing and Helen Bilton for indexing, Conal Daly and David Oliver for useful comments and challenges, and Phil Hammond for making me laugh over evidence-based policy making, for 22 consecutive nights in 2016. Special thanks to Richard Comber – thank you.

I have tried not to make mistake. The ones that remain are mine, and I will correct them if you tell me.

margaret@margaretmccartney.com
@mgtmccartney

References

INTRODUCTION
1   Campbell D. NHS 'will miss £22bn efficiency savings target', says thinktank. *Guardian*, 23 April 2015
2   Smyth C. Warning of cuts as NHS told to save extra £1.6bn. *Times*, 22 July 2016

CHAPTER 1
1   Griffiths C, Brock A. Twentieth Century Mortality Trends in England and Wales. *Health Statistics Quarterly* 2003;18:5–17
2   Pattison J, McPherson K, Blakemore C, Haberman S, et al for the Longevity Science Advisory Panel. *Life Expectancy: Past and Future Variations by Gender in England and Wales.* LSAP, 2012
3   From the archive, 5 July 1948: Creation of NHS heralds new era in British healthcare. *Guardian*, 5 July 2013
4   State Organised Medicine, Dr Charles Hill in conversation with Dr Bourne (radio interview). *Home Service*, 5 February 1943
5   The Health and Social Care Information Centre — Workforce Directorate. *General and Personal Medical Services: England: 2002–2012 as at 30 September*. HSCIC, 21 March 2013
6   Kaffash J. Average GP practice receives £136 per patient annually — less than a Sky TV subscription. *Pulse*, 12 February 2015
7   Francis G. Cash for Diagnoses. *London Review of Books* 2015;37(5):21
8   Cameron: 'Trust Me On The Future Of NHS'. *Sky News*, 7 June 2011.
9   Cameron: Trust me with the NHS. *politics.co.uk*, 8 June 2011
10 Mcpherson K. Nick Clegg challenges party leaders on NHS funding. *libdems.co.uk*, 31 March 2015
11 Shona Robinson Msp: Our commitment to our NHS
12 Labour's NHS Rescue Plan. Transcription of speech given by Ed Miliband, leader of the Labour Party, at Manchester Metropolitan University, Manchester, United Kingdom, 21 April 2015
13 Bevan A. *Democratic Values. First in the Series of Fabian Autumn Lectures 1950: Whither Socialism? Values in a Changing Civilisation (no.282)*. London: Fabian Publications, 1951.
14 McConaghie A. Soliris, the world's most expensive drug: will NICE judge it affordable? *Pharmaphorum*
15 Taylor D. Councils tendering care contracts case by case in online 'auctions'. *Guardian*, 27 August 2014
16 Swinford S. The 8,000 NHS staff on six figure salaries. *Telegraph*, 21 April 2013
17 Hautot J. Why I had to confront Andrew Lansley about the NHS. *Guardian*, 21 February 2012

CHAPTER 2
1   Ipsos MORI. NHS continues to be top issue for British voters. Ipsos MORI Political Monitor, 20 April 2015 and Quigley A. Maintaining pride in the NHS: The challenge for the new NHS Chief Exec. Ipsos MORI, 8 May 2014
2   Commission for Healthcare Audit and Inspection. Investigation into Mid Staffordshire NHS. Healthcare Commission, March 2009. and The Mid Staffordshire NHS Foundation Trust Public Inquiry. London: The Stationary Office, 6 February 2013
3   The Mid Staffordshire NHS Foundation Trust Public Inquiry. Witness statement of Dr Christopher Mitchell Turner given 22 February 2011
4   Letham K, Alisdair G, The four-hour target in NHS emergency departments - a critical review. *Emergencias* 2012 (24) 69-72
5   National Health Service. Accident and Emergency Attendances in England 2012–13. NHS,

28 January 2014.

6   Department of Health. A Short Guide to NHS Foundation Trusts

7   Butler P, Parker S. Q&A: Foundation Trusts. *Guardian*, 13 November 2002

8   University Hospitals Birmingham NHS Foundation Trust. Foundation Trust Questions and Answers.

9   http://www.politics.co.uk/reference/foundation-hospitals

10 Department of Health and The Rt Hon Jeremy Hunt MP. Francis report on Mid Staffs: Government accepts recommendations, 19 November 2013

11 Department of Health. *Hard Truths: The Journey to Putting Patients First: Volume One of the Government Response to the Mid Staffordshire NHS Foundation Trust Public Inquiry.* London, The Stationary Office, January 2014

12 Newdick C, Danbury C. Culture, compassion and clinical neglect: probity in the NHS after Mid Staffordshire. *J Med Ethics* 2015;41(12):956–962

13 Ibid.

14 Centre of Risk for Health Care Research and Practice. Case Study: Wayne Jowett

15 Anger as a fatal jab doctor freed. *BBC*, 23 September 2003

16 Gilbar P. Inadvertent intrathecal administration of vincristine: Has anything changed? *J Oncol Pharm Pract* March 2012;18(1):155–157

17 Public Administration Select Committee. Reducing the risk of untoward clinical incidents through learning. In: *Investigating clinical incidents in the NHS — Public Administration.* London, The Stationary Office, 27 March 2015

18 Gilbar P, Seger AC. Deaths reported from the accidental intrathecal administration of bortezomib. *J Oncol Pharm Pract* 2012;18:377–8

19 Ibid.

20 Medical Defence Union. Medico-legal Guide to Statutory Duty of Candour

21 House of Commons Health Committee. *After Francis: Making a Difference: Third Report of Session 2013–14.* London: The Stationary Office, 18 September 2013

22 Department of Health Strategy and External Relation Directorate/Quality Regulation/17160. *New criminal offence of ill-treatment or wilful neglect* consultation document, February 2014

23 Bradshaw P. Criminal offence of wilful neglect may undermine, rather than improve, patient safety. *BMJ Careers*, 8 April 2015

24 Heywood J. Whistleblowers

25 Brimelow A. NHS 'whistleblower demands apology and comparable job'. *BBC*, 7 March 2015 [www.bbc.co.uk/news/health-31772025] and Costello T. NHS Gagging Orders: The NHS whistleblower and the £500,000 'supergag'. *Bureau of Investigative Journalism*, 29 June 2012

26 Butler P. Great Ormond Street hospital issues apology to Baby P whistleblower. *Guardian*, 14 June 2011

CHAPTER 3

1   National Health Service. About the NHS: NHS Core Principles

2   Oliver M. Exclusive: Prime Minister David Cameron clashes with Oxfordshire County Council over cuts to frontline services. *Oxford Mail*, 11 November 2015

3   Monbiot G. David Cameron hasn't the faintest idea how deep his cuts go. This letter proves it. *Guardian*, 11 November 2015

4   Hastings A, Bailey N, Besemer K, Bramley G, Gannon M, Watkins D. *Coping with the cuts? Local government and proorer communities.* Glasgow: Joseph Rowntree Foundation, 28 November 2013

5   Ibid.

6   Commission on the Future of Health and Social Care in England. Statement by Dame Kate Barker CBE, Geoff Alltimes CBE, Lord Bichard, Baroness Sally Greengross, Sir Julian Le Grand, November 2015

7   Age UK. *Care in Crisis: What's Next for Social Care?* London: Age UK Campaigns, January

References

2014

8   Samuel M. Social care cuts damaging the health service, warn NHS finance chiefs. *communitycare.co.uk*, 22 October 2015

9   Bardsley M, Georghiou T, Chassin L, Lewis G, Steventon A, Dixon J. Overlap of hospital use and social care in older people in England. *J Health Serv Res Policy* 2012;17:133–139

10 Thorlby R. The human cost of adult social care. Nuffield Trust and The Health Foundation, 25 June 2014

11 www.theguardian.com/society/2015/jan/07/patients-hospital-elderly-bedblockers-care

12 Appleby J. I'm a healthy patient; get me out of here. *BMJ* 2016;353:i3585

13 www.nationalvoices.org.uk/sites/www.nationalvoices.org.uk/files/im_still_me.pdf

14 McCartney M. *Living with Dying*. London: Pinter & Martin, 2014, p30

15 Beswick AD, Rees K, Dieppe P, Ayis S, Gooberman-Hill R, Horwood J, Ebrahim S. Complex interventions to improve physical function and maintain independent living in elderly people: a systematic review and meta-analysis. *Lancet* 2008 Mar;371(9614):725–735

16 Age UK. Care in Crisis 2014

17 Holt-Lunstad J, Smith TB, Baker M, et al. Loneliness and social isolation as risk factors for mortality: a meta- analytic review. *Perspect Psychol Sci* 2015;10:227–37

18 Flegal KM, Kit BK, Orpana H, Graubard BI. Association of All-Cause Mortality With Overweight and Obesity Using Standard Body Mass Index Categories: A Systematic Review and Meta-analysis. *JAMA.* 2013;309(1):71–82

19 Humphries R. Social care funding and the NHS: An impending crisis? London: The King's Fund, 17 March 2011

20 NHS Confederation. Papering over the cracks: the impact of social care funding on the NHS. NHS Reform and Transition: Briefing, Issue 248, September 2012

21 D'Souza S. Preventing admission of older people to hospital. *BMJ* 2013;346:f3186

22 Appleby J. The hospital bed: on its way out? *BMJ* 2013;346

23 ones R. Bed Occupancy – don't take it lying down. *Health Service Journal*;111(5752):28–31

24 The King's Fund. The NHS in a nutshell: The number of hospital beds

25 Helm T, Doward J. Beds crisis hits NHS care for mentally ill children. *Guardian*, 31 January 2015

26 McNicoll A. 101 ways the mental health beds crisis is hitting patient care. *communitycare. co.uk*, October 16 2013

29 Shields M. 'The system failed him in the most catastrophic way' — Father's anger at mental health over son's suicide. *Eastern Daily Press*, 17 October 2013

28 Smith G, Nicholson K, Fitch C, Mynors-Wallis L for The Commission on Acute Adult Psychiatric Care. Background briefing paper: The Commission to Review the Provision of Acute Inpatient Psychiatric Care for Adults in England, Wales and Northern Ireland.

29 McNicoll A. Rise in mental health bed occupancy. *communitycare.co.uk*, June 4 2015

30 McCartney M. Well enough to work? *BMJ* 2011;342

31 Mind. Victory for welfare campaigners as government loses appeal against benefits ruling. *mind.org.uk*, 4 December 2013

32 Department for Work and Pensions. Disability Living Allowance Reform impact assessment, May 2012

33 The Consultant EU. Atos, Capita Scoop £500 Million in UK DWP Disability award

34 Gentleman A. Delays and disarray shatter lives of new disability claimants. *Guardian*, 27 January 2015

35 Butler P. Disabled payment delay unlawful, judge rules. *Guardian*, 5 June 2015

36 Garthwhaite K, Bambra C. Food poverty, welfare reform and health inequalities. In: Foster L, Brunton A, Deeming C, Haux T, eds. *In Defence of Welfare 2*, p121–3. Social Policy Association, 2015. Available at www.social-policy.org.uk/wordpress/wp-content/ uploads/2015/04/33_garthwaite-bambra.pdf. Also Rickman D, McKernan B. Sixteen of the most senseless benefit sanction decisions known to man. *Independent*, 28 October 2015

37 Written evidence submitted by Mind to the Work and Pensions Select Committee inquiry

into benefit sanctions 2014

38 Cuts in CAB funding leaving thousands with nowhere to turn for help. *citizensadvice.org. uk*, 6 September 2011

39 Get people with mental health problems off mainstream back to work schemes says Mind. *mind.org.uk*, 11 December 2014

40 United Nations Commission on Human Rights. Documentation regarding CESCR — International Covenant on Economic, Social and Cultural Rights 58 Session, 6–24 June 2016. Available at tbinternet.ohchr.org/_layouts/treatybodyexternal/SessionDetails1. aspx?SessionID=1059&Lang=en.

41 Barr B, Taylor-Robinson D, Stuckler D, Loopstra R, Reeves A, Whitehead M. 'First, do no harm': are disability assessments associated with adverse trends in mental health? A longitudinal ecological study. *J Epidemiol Community Health*, 16 November 2015

42 Lacobucci G. GPs' workload climbs as government austerity agenda bites. *BMJ* 2014;349 and Lacobucci G. GPs increasingly have to tackle patients' debt and housing problems. *BMJ* 2014;349

43 Ashworth-Hayes S. Poverty in the UK: a guide to the facts and figures. London: Full Fact, 18 August 2016

44 Oxfam. Food Poverty in the UK

45 Garthwaite K, Bambra C. Food poverty, welfare reform and health inequalities. (see 35).

46 Evidence submitted by The Trussell Trust to the Work and Pensions Select Committee inquiry into benefit sanctions

47 Taylor-Robinson D, Wickham S, Barr B. Child health at risk from welfare cuts. *BMJ* 2015;351

48 Finch D. A Poverty of information: Assessing the government's new child poverty focus and future trends. Resolution Foundation, October 7 2015

49 Taylor-Robinson D, et al. Child health at risk from welfare cuts. (see 46).

50 Childhood, Infant and Perinatal Mortality in England and Wales, 2012. Office for National Statistics, 30 January 2014

51 Faculty of Dental Surgery. The State of Children's Oral Health in England, January 2015

52 Public Health England. *National Dental Epidemiology Programme for England: Oral Health Survey of Five-Year-Old Children 2012: A report on the prevalence and severity of dental decay*. London: Public Health England, 2013

53 Rudge GM, Mohammed MA, Fillingham SC, Girling A, Sidhu K, Stevens AJ. Jiang B, ed. The combined influence of distance and neighbourhood deprivation on emergency department attendance in a large English population: a retrospective database study. *PLoS One* 2013;8(7):e67943.

54 Barnett K, Mercer SW, Norbury M, Watt G, Wyke S, Guthrie B. Epidemiology of multimorbidity and implications for health care, research, and medical education: a cross-sectional study. *Lancet* 2012 Jul 7; 380(9836):37–43

55 Charlton J, Rudisill C, Bhattarai N, Gulliford M. Impact of deprivation on occurrence, outcomes and health care costs of people with multiple morbidity. *J Health Serv Res Policy* 2013 Oct;18(4):215–223

56 Office for National Statistics. *Inequality in Healthy Life Expectancy at Birth by National Deciles of Area Deprivation: England, 2009–11*. Available at www.ons.gov.uk/ons/rel/ disability-and-health-measurement/inequality-in-healthy-life-expectancy-at-birth-by-national-deciles-of-area-deprivation--england/2009-11/stb---inequality-in-hle.html.

57 UCL Institute of Health Equity. 'Fair Society Healthy Lives' (The Marmot Review)

58 Tudor Hart J. The Inverse Care Law. *Lancet* 1971 Feb;297(7696):405–412

59 *The Black Report 1980*. Available from Socialist Health Association

60 Marmot M. The richer you are, the better your health — and how this can be changed. *Guardian*, 11 September 2015

61 UCL Institute of Health Equity. *Health Inequalities Evidence Review*. London: Public Health England, September 2014

62 Hough J, Rice B. *Providing personalised support to rough sleepers*. York: Joseph Rowntree

References

Foundation, October 2010

63 McCartney M. Cash as a treatment for poverty. *BMJ* 2015;351:h5752

64 Forget EL. *The Town with No Poverty: Using Health Administration Data to Revisit Outcomes of a Canadian Guaranteed Annual Income Field Experiment.* Manitoba: University of Manitoba, February 2011

65 Teed P, McCartney M. Are Medical organisations leading by example on pay? *BMJ* 2015;351:h5387

66 Harris J, Domokos J. Hospital cleaners stage one-day strike for London living wage. *Guardian*, 21 March 2016and Hastings A, Bailey N, Bramley G, Gannon M, Watkins D. *The cost of the cuts: the impact on local government and poorer communities.* York: Joseph Rowntree Foundation, 10 March 2015

67 Sure Start: The Development of an Early Intervention Programme for Young Children in the United Kingdom. *Children & Society* 1999;139(4):257–264

68 Abrams F. Sure Start: Are children really benefitting? *BBC*, 12 July 2011

69 The National Evaluation of Sure Start Team. *The impact of Sure Start Local Programmes on five year olds and their families.* London: Department for Education, November 2010

70 Hutchings J, Bywater T, Daley D, Gardner F, Whitaker C, Jones K, Eames C, Edwards R. Parenting intervention in Sure Start services for children at risk of developing conduct disorder: pragmatic randomised controlled trial. *BMJ* 2007;334:678

71 The National Evaluation of Sure Start Team. *The impact of Sure Start Local Programmes on five year olds and their families.* (see 68).

72 McVeigh T. Sure Start children's centres face worst year of budget cuts, says charity. *Guardian*, 12 October 2014

73 Torjesen I. Austerity cuts are eroding benefits of Sure Start children's centres. *BMJ* 2016; 352:i335

74 Sammons P, Hall J, Smees R, et al and University of Oxford. Research report: The impact of children's centres: studying the effects of children's centres in promoting better outcomes for young children and their families. Department for Education, December 2015

75 Wakefield MA, Germain D, Durkin SJ. How does increasingly plainer cigarette packaging influence adult smokers' perceptions about brand image? An experimental study. *Tob Control* 2008 Dec; 17(6): 416–421

76 Limb M. Government has lost 'credibility on public health' for inaction on cigarettes and alcohol, campaigners say. *BMJ* 2013;346:f3024

77 Doward J. Conservative election guru Lynton Crosby lobbied minister over tobacco. *Guardian*, 6 September 2014

78 Gornall J. Tickets to Glyndebourne or the Ocal? Big tobacco's bid to woo parlimentarians, *BMJ* 2015:350:h2509

79 Wakefield MA, Hayes L, Durkin S, Borland R. Introduction effects of the Australian plain packaging policy on adult smokers: a cross-sectional study. *BMJ Open* 2013;3:e003175

80 Scollo M, Zacher M, Durkin S, Wakefield M. Early evidence about the predicted unintended consequences of standardised packaging of tobacco products in Australia: a cross-sectional study of the place of purchase, regular brands and use of illicit tobacco. *BMJ Open* 2014;4:e005873

81 Australian Government Department of Health. Tobacco Control key facts and figures, 29 June 2016

82 Report of the independent review undertaken by Sir Cyril Chantler: Standardised packaging of tobacco, April 2014. Available at www.kcl.ac.uk/health/10035-TSO-2901853-Chantler-Review-ACCESSIBLE.PDF.

83 Health and Social Care Information Centre. Statistics on Smoking: England 2014. HSCIC, 8 October 2014

84 Hatchard JL, Fooks GJ, Evans-Reeves KA, Ulucanlar S, Gilmore AB. A critical evaluation of the volume, relevance and quality of evidence submitted by the tobacco industry to oppose standardised packaging of tobacco products. *BMJ Open* 2014;4:e003757

85 Ram A. Tobacco giants launch UK plain packaging challenge. *Financial Times*, 8

December 2015

86 Prescott CA, Caldwell CB, Carey G, Vogler GP, Trumbetta SL, Gottesman II. The Washington University Twin Study of alcoholism. *Am J Med Genet B Neuropsychiatr Genet* 2005 Apr 5;134B(1):48–55 [www.ncbi.nlm.nih.gov/pubmed/15704214] and Royal College of Psychiatrists. Alcoholism data

87 Fone DL, Farewell DM, White J, Lyons RA, Dunstan FD. Socioeconomic patterning of excess alcohol consumption and binge drinking: a cross-sectional study of multilevel associations with neighbourhood deprivation. *BMJ Open* 2013;3:e002337 National Health Service. Binge Drinking

88 The King's Fund. What's going on in A&E? The key questions answered, 3 March 2016

89 Parkinson K, Newbury-Birch D, Phillipson A, et al. Prevalence of alcohol related attendance at an inner city emergency department and its impact: a dual prospective and retrospective cohort study. *Emerg Med J* Published Online First: 23 December 2015

90 Currie C, Davies A, Blunt I, Ariti C, Bardsley M for Nuffield Trust. *Alcohol-specific Activity in Hospitals in England*. London: Nuffield Trust, December 2015

91 Warner J, Minghao H, Gmel G, Rehm J. Can Legislation Prevent Debauchery? Mother Gin and Public Health in 18th-century England. *American Journal of Public Health* 2001 Mar;91(3):375–384

92 Stockwell T, Auld M C, Zhao J, Martin G, (2012), Does minimum pricing reduce alcohol consumption? The experience of a Canadian province. *Addiction* 2012 May;107:912–920

93 Stockwell T, Zhao J, Marzell M, Gruenewald P, Macdonald S, Ponicki WR, Martin G. Relationships Between Minimum Alcohol Pricing and Crime During Privatization of a Canadian Government Alcohol Monopoly. *Journal of Studies on Alcohol and Drugs* 2015;76(4):628–634

94 Stockwell T, Zhao J, Martin G, Macdonald S, Vallance K, Treno A, Ponicki W, Tu A, Buxton J. Minimum Alcohol Prices and Outlet Densities in British Columbia, Canada: Estimated Impacts on Alcohol-Attributable Hospital Admissions. *American Journal of Public Health* 2013;103(11)

95 Zhao J, Stockwell T, Martin G, Macdonald S, Vallance K, Treno A, Ponicki W R, Tu A, Buxton J. The relationship between minimum alcohol prices, outlet densities and alcohol-attributable deaths in British Columbia, 2002–09. *Addiction* 2013; 108: 1059–1069

96 Stockwell T, Thomas G for Institute of Alcohol Studies. *Is alcohol too cheap in the UK? The case for setting a Minimum Unit Price for alcohol. Institute of Alcohol Studies*, April 2013

97 Griffith R, Leicester A, O'Connell M for Institute of Fiscal Studies. Briefing Note BN138: *Price-based measures to reduce alcohol consumption*. Economic and Social Research Council, March 2013

98 Chalmers J. Alcohol minimum unit pricing and socioeconomic status. *Lancet* 2014 May;383(9929)1616–1617

99 Proposed minimum alcohol price law is published. *BBC*, 15 July 2015

100 Carrell S. Minimum alcohol price in Scotland breaches EU law, court rules. *Guardian*, 23 December 2015

101 Scottish Government. Minimum Unit Pricing

102 House of Commons Health Committee. *Alcohol: First Report of Session 2009–10 Volume 1*. London: The Stationary Office, 8 January

103 Department of Health. Public Health Responsibility Deal launches new alcohol pledge, 23 March 2012

104 Health and Social Care Information Centre. Statistics on Alcohol: England 2015. HSCIC, 25 June 2015

105 *The Government's Alcohol Strategy*. London: The Stationary Office, 22 March 2012

106 Gornall J. Under the influence. *BMJ* 2014;348:f7646

107 Minimum alcohol pricing plan 'may breach EU law'. *BBC*, September 23 2015

108 National Institute for Health and Care Excellence. *NICE Indicators Programme: Consultation on potential new indicators*. NICE, 2016

109 Millett D. Interview with Professor Dame Sally Davies: Fighting the UK's public health

References

crisis. *gponline.com*, 23 May 2014

110 i0.wp.com/www.carlheneghan.com/wp-content/uploads/2013/08/Untitled.png.

111 Furber CM, McGowan L, Bower P, Kontopantelis E, Quenby S, Lavender T. Antenatal interventions for reducing weight in obese women for improving pregnancy outcome. *Cochrane Database of Systematic Reviews* 2013; Issue 1 Art. No.: CD009334

112 Waters E, de Silva-Sanigorski A, Burford BJ, Brown T, Campbell KJ, Gao Y, Armstrong R, Prosser L, Summerbell CD. Interventions for preventing obesity in children. *Cochrane Database of Systematic Reviews* 2011, Issue 12. Art. No.: CD001871

113 Bray GA. Some historical aspects of drug treatment for obesity. Pharmacotherapy of Obesity. In: *Milestones in Drug Therapy*:11–19. Switzerland: Birkhäuser Verlag, 2008

114 Medicines and Healthcare Products Regulatory Agency. Sibutramine: suspension of EU licences recommended. Drug Safety Update Feb 2010, Vol 3 Issue 7: 7a

115 Colquitt JL, Pickett K, Loveman E, Frampton GK. Surgery for Obesity: What are the effects of weight loss (bariatric) surgery for overweight or obese adults? *Cochrane Database of Systematic Reviews*, 8 August 2014

116 Department of Health. *The Public Health Responsibility Deal*, March 2011

117 Department of Health. Calories to be capped and cut (press release), 24 March 2012

118 Knai C, Petticrew M, Durand A, Eastmure E, James L, Mehrotra A, Scott C, Mays N. Has a public–private partnership resulted in action on healthier diets in England? An analysis of the Public Health Responsibility Deal food pledges. *Food Policy* 2015 Jul; 54:1–10

119 Kantar Worldpanel Usage. Salt, sugar, fat: A consumer's eye view

120 Department for Environment, Food & Rural Affairs. Detailed annual statistics on family food and drink purchases, 13 December 2012

121 Durand MA, Petticrew M, Goulding L, Eastmure E, Knai C, Mays N. An evaluation of the Public Health Responsibility Deal: Informants' experiences and views of the development, implementation and achievements of a pledge-based, public–private partnership to improve population health in England. *Health Policy*;119(11):1506–1514

122 McCartney M. Is Coca-Cola's antiobesity scheme the real thing? *BMJ* 2014;349:g4340

123 Associated Press. Coca-Cola discloses it spent $119m on health research over five years. *Guardian*, 22 September 2015

124 Archer E, Pavela G, Lavie CJ. The Inadmissibility of What We Eat in America and NHANES Dietary Data in Nutrition and Obesity Research and the Scientific Formulation of National Dietary Guidelines. *Mayo Clinic Proceedings*;90(7):911–926

125 Hu FB. Resolved: there is sufficient scientific evidence that decreasing sugar-sweetened beverage consumption will reduce the prevalence of obesity and obesity-related diseases. *Obes Rev* 2013 Aug;14(8):606–19

126 ASA Ruling on Coca-Cola Great Britain, 27 April 2011. Available at www.asa.org.uk/ Rulings/Adjudications/2011/4/Coca_Cola-Great-Britain/TF_ADJ_50308.aspx.

127 Basu S, McKee M, Galea G, Stuckler D. Relationship of soft drink consumption to global overweight, obesity, and diabetes: a cross-national analysis of 75 countries. *Am J Public Health* 2013 Nov;103(11):2071–7

128 Colchero MA, Popkin BM, Rivera JA, Ng SW. Beverage purchases from stores in Mexico under the excise tax on sugar sweetened beverages: observational study. *BMJ* 2016;352:h6704

129 Cabrera Escobar MA, Lennert Veerman J, Tollman SM, Bertram MY, Hofman KJ. Evidence that a tax on sugar sweetened beverages reduces the obesity rate: a meta-analysis. *BMC Public Health* 2013; 13:1072

130 Gornall J. Sugar: spinning a web of influence. *BMJ* 2015;350:h231

131 HM Treasury. Policy paper: Budget 2016, March 2016. Available at www.gov.uk/ government/publications/budget-2016-documents/budget-2016.

132 Daneshkhu S, Neville S, Pickard J. Sugar tax attacked by soft-drink makers after Budget. *Financial Times*, 16 March 2016

133 McCartney M. Can doctors fix cold homes? *BMJ* 2015;350:h231

134 Howden-Chapman P1, Pierse N, Nicholls S, Gillespie-Bennett J, Viggers H, Cunningham

M, Phipps R, Boulic M, Fjällström P, Free S, Chapman R, Lloyd B, Wickens K, Shields D, Baker M, Cunningham C, Woodward A, Bullen C, Crane J. Effects of improved home heating on asthma in community dwelling children: randomised controlled trial. *BMJ* 2008 Sep 23;337:a1411

135 Thomson H, Thomas S, Sellstrom E, Petticrew M. Housing improvement as an investment to improve health. *Cochrane Database of Systematic Reviews*, 28 February 2013

CHAPTER 4

1   Greenstone G. The history of bloodletting. *BCMJ* 2010 Jan, Feb;52(1):12–14

2   Parapia LA. History of bloodletting by phlebotomy. *British Journal of Haematology* 2008;143:490–495

3   Warner JH. Therapeutic explanation and the Edinburgh bloodletting controversy: two perspectives on the medical meaning of science in the mid-nineteenth century. *Med Hist* 1980;24(3):254 [

4   Ibid, p256.

5   House of Commons Health Committee. *The Influence of the Pharmaceutical Industry: Fourth Report of Session 2004–2005: Volume II.* London: The Stationary Office; 26 April 2005.

6   Milne I. Who was James Lind, and what exactly did he achieved? JLL Bulletin: Commentaries on the history of treatment evaluation

7   The James Lind Library

8   Chalmers I. Reducing waste in deciding what research to do. Report of NIHR Trainees Meeting, Leeds, 26 November 2013

9   NHS Confederation. Key statistics on the NHS, 2 September 2016

10 Testing Treatments Interactive. Key Concepts for critical thinking about treatment claims

11 Kenealy T, Arroll B. Antibiotics for the common cold and acute purulent rhinitis. *Cochrane Database of Systematic Reviews* 2013, Issue 6, Art No. CD000247

12 Mistry K. Determining the Effects of desPLEX. *Yale Scientific*, 26 February 2009

13 Watkins Smith O. Diethylstilbestrol in the prevention and treatment of complications of pregnancy. *Obstetrical & Gynecological Survey* 1949 Apr;4(2):190–191

14 Dieckmann WJ, Davis ME, Rynkiewicz LM, Pottinger RE. Does the administration of diethylstilbestrol during pregnancy have therapeutic value? *Am J Obstet Gynecol* 1953 Nov;66(5):1062–81

15 National Cancer Institute. Diethylstilbestrol (DES) and Cancer

16 Kenter MJH, et al. Establishing risk of human experimentation with drugs: lessons from TGN1412. *Lancet*;368(9544):1387–1391

17 Goodyear M. Learning from the TGN1412 trial. *BMJ* 2006;332:677

18 Suntharalingam G, Perry MR, Ward S, Brett SJ, Castello-Cortes A, Brunner MD, Panoskaltsis N. Cytokine Storm in a Phase 1 Trial of the Anti-CD28 Monoclonal Antibody TGN1412. *N Engl J Med* 2006;355:1018–1028

19 Kenter MJH, Cohen AF. Establishing risk of human experimentation with drugs: lessons from TGN1412. *Lancet* 2006;368(9544):1387–1391

20 Chalmers I. TGN1412 and *The Lancet*'s solicitation of reports of phase I trials. *Lancet*;368(9554):2206–2207

21 Dyer O. Experimental drug that injured UK volunteers resumes in human trials. *BMJ* 2015;350:h1831

22 Savulescu J, Spriggs M. The hexamethonium asthma study and the death of a normal volunteer in research. *J Med Ethics* 2002;28:3–4

23 The story of the Cochrane logo

24 Altman DG. The scandal of poor medical research. *BMJ* 1994;308:283

25 AllTrials

26 Anderson ML, Chiswell K, Peterson ED, Tasneem A, Topping J, Califf RM. Compliance with Results Reporting at ClinicalTrials.gov. *N Engl J Med* 2015;372:1031–1039

27 House of Commons Committee of Public Accounts. *Access to clinical trial information and*

the stockpiling of Tamiflu: Thirty-fifth Report of Session 2013–14. London: The Stationary Office, 3 January 2014

28 British Medical Journal. Tamiflu data: Who saw what when

29 House of Commons Committee of Public Accounts. *Access to clinical trial information and the stockpiling of Tamiflu.* (see 27).

30 Dryden R, Williams B, McCowen C, Themessl-Huber M. What do we know about who does and does not attend general health checks? Finding from a narrative scoping review. *BMC Public Health* 2012;12:723

31 McCartney M. Where's the evidence for NHS health checks? *BMJ* 2013;347:F5834

32 Johnson F, Beeken RJ, Croker H, Wardle J. Do weight perceptions among obese adults in Great Britain match clinical definitions? Analysis of cross-sectional surveys from 2007 and 2012. *BMJ Open* 2014;4(11):e005561

33 National Obesity Forum. *State of the Nation's Waistline.* 2014.

34 Blackburn M, Stathi A, Keogh E, Eccleston C. Raising the topic of weight in general practice: perspectives of GPs and primary care nurses. *BMJ Open* 2015;5(8):e008546

35 Cavill, N; Hillsdon M; Anstiss T; *Brief interventions for weight management.* Oxford: National Obesity Observatory, 2011 https://www.phc.ox.ac.uk/events/oxford-primary-care-clinical-update-for-gps-1/jebb.pdf

36 The men who made us thin: the evidence. *carlheneghan.com*, 14 August 2013

37 Lewis E. Why there's no point telling me to lose weight. *BMJ* 2015;350:G6845

38 Robinson E, Hunger JM, Daly M. Perceived weight status and risk of weight gain across life in US and UK adults. *International Journal of Obesity* 2015;39:1721–1726

39 Heleno B, Thomsen MF, Rodrigues DS, Jørgensen KJ, Brodersen J. Quantification of harms in cancer screening trials: literature review. *BMJ* 2013;347:f5334

40 National Institute for Health and Care Excellence. Clinical Guideline: Cardiovascular disease: risk assessment and reduction, including lipid modification. NICE, July 2014 (updated July 2016)

41 National Institute for Health and Care Excellence. NICE recommends wider use of statins for prevention of CVD

42 National Institute for Health and Care Excellence. Costing report: Lipid modification: Implementing the NICE guideline on lipid modification (CG181). Manchester, NICE, July 2014

43 Campbell D. Price to be written on NHS-prescribed medicine costing more than £20. *Guardian*, 1 July 2015

44 Watt N. Patients could be charged for missed NHS appointments, says Jeremy Hunt. *Guardian*, 3 July 2015

45 Department of Health. *Reducing missed hospital appointments using text messages: a zero cost way to reduce missed hospital* appointments – research and analysis. Available at www.gov.uk/government/publications/reducing-missed-hospital-appointments-using-text-messages.

46 Hallsworth M, Berry D, Sanders M, Sallis A, King D, et al. Stating Appointment Costs in SMS Reminders Reduces Hospital Appointments: Findings from Two Randomised Trials. *PLoS ONE* 2015;10(9):e0137306

47 www.gov.uk/government/uploads/system/uploads/attachment_data/file/448466/NHS_Constitution_WEB.pdf

CHAPTER 5

1 Factcheck: David Cameron's broken promises. *Channel 4 News*, 17 March 2015

2 "The end of the NHS as we know it"? A guide to the Health and Social Care Act. London: Full Fact, 28 March 2013

3 Conservative 2015 Manifesto

4 Roberts SE, Thorne K, Akbari A, Samuel DG, Williams JG. Mortality following Stroke, the Weekend Effect and Related Factors: Record Linkage Study. Dalal K, ed. *PLoS ONE* 2015;10(6):e0131836

5   British Medical Association. European Working Time Directive: Junior doctors FAQ. BMA, 14 May 2012 (updated 30 June 2016)

6   Triggle N. Jeremy Huant: Doctors 'must work weekends'. *BBC*, 16 July 2015

7   Triggle N. Junior doctors row: 98% vote in favour of strikes. *BBC*, 19 November 2015

8   Letters: Junior doctors have our consultants' full support in this dispute with Jeremy Hunt. *Guardian*, 13 November 2015

9   Royal College of General Practitioners. RCGP demands 'cast iron guarantee' on junior doctors' contract

10 Lacobucci G. Up to a quarter of GP out-of-hours shifts left unfilled. *Pulsetoday.co.uk*, 18 January 2012

11 National Health Service. Agency controls significantly reduce NHS spend on agency staff. NHS Improvement, 9 May 2016

12 Public Accounts Committee. Sustainability and financial performance of acute hospital trusts inquiry, 15 March 2016

13 Department of Health, Commissioning Development Directorate, Primary Medical Care. *Guidance: GP Extended Hours Access Scheme Directed Enhanced Service–1 April 2011 to 31 March 2012*. London: The Stationary Office, 4 April 2011

14 NHS England. Prime Minister's GP Access Fund

15 Bostock N. DH to press ahead with seven-day GP access plans. *gponline.com*, 30 October 2015

16 Ford JA, Jones AP, Wong G, Steel N. Weekend opening in primary care: analysis of the General Practice Patient Survey. *Br J Gen Pract* Nov 2015

17 Lind S. GP seven-day pilot schemes being abandoned in blow to Conservatives' access drive. *pulsetoday.co.uk*, 7 May 2015

18 Lind S. Half of PM's seven-day GP access pilots have cut opening hours. *pulsetoday.co.uk*, 29 September 2015

19 Rosen R for Nuffield Trust in partnership with NHS England. *Meeting need of fuelling demand?: Improved access to primary care and supply-induced demand*. London: Nuffield Trust, June 2014

20 Kenny C, Raffish J, Matthews-King A. Revealed: Sixty GP practices across the country facing imminent closure. *pulsetoday.co.uk*, 3 July 2014

21 Freeman G, Hughes J. *Continuity of Care and the Patient Experience: An Inquiry into the Quality of General Practice*. London: The King's Fund, 2010

22 Wintour P. Jeremy Hunt: I cannot negotiate on manifesto promise of 24-hour NHS. *Guardian*, 4 November 2015

23 Thomas CJ, Smith RP, Uzoigwe CE, Braybrooke JR. The weekend effect. *Bone Joint J* 2014;96–B:373–8

24 Jeremy Hunt: 'We have 6,000 avoidable deaths every year' (recorded interview). *BBC*, 16 July 2015

35 Freemantle N, Daniel R, McNulty D, Rosser D, Bennett S, Keogh BE, et al. Increased mortality associated with weekend hospital admission: a case for expanded seven day services? *BMJ* 2015; 315:h4596

26 Meacock R, Anselmi L, Kristensen SR, Doran T, Sutton M. Higher mortality rates amongst emergency patients admitted to hospital at weekends reflect a lower probability of admission. *J Health Serv Res Policy* May 2016

27 Meacock R, Doran T, Sutton M. What are the Costs and Benefits of Providing Comprehensive Seven-day Services for Emergency Hospital Admissions? *Health Econ* Aug 2015;24(8):907–12

28 House of Commons debate on Junior Doctors' Contract record, 25 April 2016. Available at hansard.parliament.uk/commons/2016-04-25/debates/16042516000001/JuniorDoctorsContracts.

29 Letter from Chair of UK Statistics Authority, Sir Andrew Dilnot CBE, in reference to statement made regarding British Medical Journal article on mortality in hospitals on weekends. Available at www.statisticsauthority.gov.uk/wp-content/uploads/2015/12/

References

images-letterfromsirandrewdilnottocd03121_tcm97-45051.pdf and Ruiz M, Bottle A, Aylin PP. The Global Comparators project: international comparison of 30-day in-hospital mortality by day of the week. *BMJ Qual Saf* 2015

30   Lilford RJ, Chen Y. The ubiquitous weekend effect: moving past proving it exists to clarifying what causes it. *BMJ Qual Saf* 2015

31   House of Commons debate record, 28 October 2015

32   Craven D. The statistical sins of Jeremy Hunt. *BMJ* 2015;351:h6358

33   Le Couteur DG, Doust J, Creasey H, Brayne C. Political drive to screen for pre-dementia: not evidence based and ignores the harms of diagnosis. *BMJ* 2013;347:f5125

34   Ibid.

35   Burns A, Twomey P, Barrett E, Harwood D, Cartmell N, Cohen D, Findlay D, Gupta S, Twomey C. *Dementia diagnosis and management: A brief pragmatic resource for general practitioners.* NHS England, 14 January 2015

36   GPs to be paid £55 for each dementia diagnosis. *BBC*, 22 October 2014 [www.bbc.co.uk/news/health-29718618] and GPs to be paid for dementia diagnosis. *alzheimersresearchuk. org*, 22 October 2014

37   Department of Health. Dementia diagnosis to be overhauled (press release), 15 May 2013

38   Price C. GPs to be paid £55 for every dementia diagnosis under new identification scheme. *pulsetoday.co.uk*, 21 October 2014

39   Price C. Cash for dementia diagnoses intended to cover GP costs, Stevens says. *pulsetoday. co.uk*, 29 October 2014 [

40   Department of Health. Dementia diagnosis to be overhauled. (see 37).

41   Burns A, Twomey P, et al. *Dementia diagnosis and management.* (see 35).

42   Price C. Dementia DES had little impact on number of patients diagnosed. *pulsetoday. co.uk*, 30 July 2014

43   Alzheimer's Society. Dementia UK: Update

44   The Telegraph. 'Dementia map': How diagnosis rates vary across England [www.telegraph. co.uk/news/health/news/10482464/Dementia-map-how-diagnosis-rates-vary-across-England.html].

45   Brunet M. Dementia diagnosis targets: a problem of scale? *Guardian*, 16 October 2014

46   Price C. Expert urges GPs to take dementia DES. *pulsetoday.co.uk*, 30 April 2013

47   Stirling A. GPs hit by widespread complaints from patients 'unhappy' over dementia screening. *pulsetoday.co.uk*, 22 November 2013

48   Price C. Dementia DES had little impact on number of patients diagnosed. (see 42).

49   Matthews FE, et al. A two-decade comparison of prevalence of dementia in individuals aged 65 years and older from three geographical areas of England: results of the Cognitive Function and Ageing Study I and II. *Lancet* Oct 2013;382(9902):1405–1412

50   Bell S, Harkness K, Dickson JM, Blackburn D. A diagnosis for £55: what is the cost of government initiatives in dementia case finding. *Age and Ageing* 2015

51   Briefing on the 2016/17 GMS contract changes

52   Select Committee on Public Accounts. Memorandum submitted by the British Medical Association: The value of general practice

53   Average GP pay rises to £106,000. *BBC*, 29 November 2006

54   National Audit Office. *NHS Pay Modernisation: New Contracts for General Practice Services in England.* London: The Stationary Office, 25 February 2008

55   Doran T, et al for National Primary Care Research and Development Centre. Quality and Outcomes Framework Analysis (QOFa) projects [www.population-health.manchester. ac.uk/primarycare/npcrdc-archive/archive/ProjectDetail.cfm/ID/157.htm].

56   Swinglehurst D, Greenhaigh T, Roberts C. Computer templates in chronic disease management: ethnographic case study in general practice. *BMJ* 2012;2(6):e001754

57   Clinical Practice Research Datalink

58   www.ingentaconnect.com/content/bcs/ipc/2004/00000012/00000002/ art00003?crawler=true

59   Silverman J. Doctors' non-verbal behaviour in consultations: look at the patient before you

look at the computer. *Br J Gen Pract* 1 Feb 2010;60(571):76–78

60 Newman W, Button G, Cairns P. Pauses in doctor-patient conversation during computer use: The design significance of their durations and accompanying topic changes. *Int J. Human-Computer Studies* 2010;68:398–402

61 Bensing JM, Tromp F, van Dulmen S, van den Brink-Muinen A, Verheul W, Schellevis FG. Shifts in doctor-patient communication between 1986 and 2002: a study of videotaped General Practice consultations with hypertension patients. *BMC Family Practice* 2006;7:62

62 Ratanawongsa N, Barton JL, Lyles CR, et al. Association Between Clinician Computer Use and Communication With Patients in Safety-Net Clinics. *JAMA Intern Med* 2016;176(1):125–128

63 Doran T, Kontopantelis E, Valderas JM, Campbell S, Roland M, Salisbury C, Reeves D. Effect of financial incentives on incentivised and non-incentivised clinical activities: longitudinal analysis of data from the UK Quality and Outcomes Framework. *BMJ* 2011;342:d3590

64 Campbell SM, McDonald R, Lester H. The experience of pay for performance in English family practice: A qualitative study. *Ann Fam Med* 1 May 2008;6(3):228–234

65 National Institute for Health and Care Excellence. NICE Guidance: Caesarean Section. NICE, November 2011 (updated August 2012)

66 Johnson EM, Rehavi MM. Physicians treating physicians: information and incentives in childbirth. New Haven: Yale University Department of Economics, April 2013

67 Department of Health. Personalised GP care will bring back old-fashioned family doctors (press release), 15 November 2013

68 'Outdated' QOF GP payment system scrapped in Scotland. *BBC*, 1 October 2015

69 British Medical Association. QOF Guidance. BMA, 23 May 2012

70 Office for National Statistics. *Compendium: Adult Smoking Habits in Great Britain, 2013*. ONS, 25 November 2014

71 Fairbrother G, Hanson KL, Friedman S, Butts GC. The impact of physician bonuses, enhanced fees, and feedback on childhood immunization coverage rates. *American Journal of Public Health* 1999;89(2):171–175

72 Collings JS. General Practice in England today: A reconnaissance. *Lancet* 25 March 1950;255(6604):555

73 Dusheiko M, Gravelle H, Hole A, Sivey P. Incentivising prevention by general practitioners: some research possibilities

74 Harrison MJ, Dusheiko M, Sutton M, Gravelle H, Doran T, Roland M. Effect of a national primary care pay for performance scheme on emergency hospital admissions for ambulatory care sensitive conditions: controlled longitudinal study. *BMJ* 2014;349:g6423

75 Kontopantelis E, Springate DA, Ashworth M, Webb RT, Buchan IE, Doran T. Investigating the relationship between quality of primary care and premature mortality in England: a spatial whole-population study. *BMJ* 2015;350:h904

76 Campbell SM, Reeves D, Kontopantelis E, Sibbald B, Roland M. Effects of pay for performance on the quality of primary care in England. *N Engl J Med* 2009;361:368–378

77 NHS England. *Enhanced Service Specification: Avoiding unplanned admissions: proactive case finding and patient review for vulnerable people 2015/16*. NHS England, 23 March 2015

78 Huntley AL, Thomas R, Mann M, Huws D, Elwyn G, Paranjothy S, Purdy S. Is case management effective in reducing the risk of unplanned hospital admissions for older people? A systematic review and meta-analysis. *Family Practice* 2013;30(3):266–275

79 NHS England. *Enhanced Service Specification: Avoiding unplanned admissions: proactive case finding and patient review for vulnerable people 2015/16*. NHS England, 23 March 2015

80 State Organised Medicine, Dr Charles Hill in conversation with Dr Bourne (radio interview). *Home Service*, 5 February 1943

81 Letters: Should GPs be paid to reduce unnecessary referrals? *BMJ* 2015;351:h6593

82 Langdon C, Peckham S. The use of financial incentives to help improve health outcomes: is

the quality and outcomes framework fit for purpose? A systematic review. *J Public Health* 2014;36(2):251–258

83 Kontopantelis E, Springate DA, Ashworth M, Webb RT, Buchan IE, Doran T. Investigating the relationship between quality of primary care and premature mortality in England: a spatial whole-population study. *BMJ* 2015;350:h904

84 "There is insufficient evidence to support or not support the use of financial incentives to improve the quality of primary healthcare. Implementation should proceed with caution and incentive schemes should be carefully designed and evaluated" Scott A, Sivey P, Ait Ouakrim D, Willenberg L, Naccarella L, Furler J, Young D. The effect of financial incentives on the quality of health care provided by primary care physicians. *Cochrane Database of Systematic Reviews* 2011, Issue 9. Art. No.: CD008451

85 www.conservatives.com/~/media/files/green%20papers/health_policy_paper.ashx?dl=true

86 Letham K, Gray A. The four-hour target in the NHS emergency departments: a critical comment. *Emergencias* 2012;24:69–72

87 Huber N. Politicians must stop encouraging 'consumerist' patient behaviour, concludes A&E study. *pulsetoday.co.uk*, 7 October 2015

88 Bevan G, Hood C. Have targets improved performance in the English NHS? *BMJ* 2006;332:419 [www.bmj.com/content/332/7538/419] and Donnelly L. Ambulances referred by NHS 111 service deliberately delayed under secret trust policy, inquiry finds. *Telegraph*, 28 February 2016

89 Donnelly L. Ambulances referred by NHS 111 service deliberately delayed under secret trust policy, inquiry finds. (see 88).

90 www.conservatives.com/~/media/files/green%20papers/health_policy_paper.ashx?dl=true

91 Donnelly L. The man with a mission to heal the health service. *Telegraph*, 20 December 2013

92 Junjua A. *Leadership vacancies in the NHS: What can be done about them?* London: The King's Fund, December 2014

93 Conservative Party NHS proposals. *"The patient will see you now, doctor": How the next Conservative Government will create an NHS personal to all.*

94 Beckford M. Hospitals told to publish surgery results in 'open source' NHS. *Telegraph*, 21 March 2011

95 www.rcseng.ac.uk/media/medianews/cardiac-surgeons-call-for-greater-transparency-and-access-to-information-for-nhs-patients

96 Renal Association. History of the UK Renal Industry

97 Clinical Practice Research Datalink

98 Department of Health. Greater choice for NHS patients across the country (press release), 11 October 2011

99 Topol EJ. Failing the public health: Rofecoxib, Merck, and the FDA. *N Engl J Med* Oct 2004;351:1707–1709

100 Waxman HA. The lessons of Vioxx: drug safety and sales. *N Engl J Med* June 2005;352:2576–2578

101 Porter M. League tables, Nits, Feeling the cold, Language–Surrogate marker on *Inside Health*, BBC Radio 4, 16 September 2015

102 Parent-led tool opens up NHS children's heart surgery data to families. London: University College London, 21 June 2016

102 NHS in crisis: Health Secretary Jeremy Hunt answers your questions. *Independent*, 10 October 2014

CHAPTER 6

1 Reynolds L, Attaran A, Hervey T, McKee M. Competition-based reform of the National Health Service in England: a one-way street? *Int J Health Serv* 2012;42(2):213–7

2 Lister J. In defiance of the evidence: conservatives threaten to "reform" away England's National Health Service. *Int J Health Serv* 2012;42(1):137–55

3 Propper C, Burgess S, Gossage D. *Competition and Quality: Evidence from the NHS*

Internal Market 1991–1999. Bristol: University of Bristol Department of Economics, May 2003.

4 Timmins N for The Institute for Government and The King's Fund. *Never Again? The story of the Health and Social Care Act 2012.* London: The King's Fund, 2012

5 Horton E, Davis J, Tomlinson J. Lancet editor and doctors write: The fight for our NHS goes on. *redpepper.org.uk*, March 2012

6 McLellan A, Middleton J, Godlee F. Lansley's NHS "reforms". *BMJ* 2012;344e709

7 Watt N, Ramesh R. Health reforms could damage NHS, warns draft risk register. *Guardian*, 26 March 2012

8 Norman Tebbit: Don't let David Cameron destroy our NHS. *Mirror*, 27 January 2012

9 Charlesworth A, Smith J, Thorlby R for Nuffield Trust. *The coalition Government's Health and social care reforms:2010–2015.* London: Nuffield Trust, 8 May 2015

10 Borland S, White J. What utter blindness! Mail probe reveals how three in four NHS trusts deny life-changing cataract surgery to thousands. *Daily* Mail, 29 July 2016

11 Nuffield Trust. UK health spending as a share of GDP

12 The King's Fund. The NHS in a nutshell: Health care spending compared to other countries

13 Stone J. The number of doctors applying to work abroad surged by 1,000 per cent on the day Jeremy Hunt imposed new contract. *Independent*, 17 February 2016

14 Campbell D. Jeremy Hunt raises doubts about long-term future of free NHS. *Guardian*, 16 July 2015

15 Adam Smith Institute. Kate Andrews discusses charging for missed GP appointments on Sky News

16 Borland S, White J. What utter blindness! (see 10).

17 Naylor C, Curry Natasha, Holder H, Ross S, Marshall L, Tait E. *Clinical Commissioning Groups: Supporting Improvement in General Practice?* London: The King's Fund, 2013

18 Dixon J, Glennerster H. What do we know about fundholding in general practice? *BMJ* 1995;311:727

19 Lawson N. *The View from No. 11: Memoirs of a Tory Radical.* London: Bantam Press, 1992, p618.

20 Kay A. The abolition of the GP fundholding scheme: a lesson in evidence-based policy making. *B J of Gen Pract* February 2002; pp141–144

21 Smith RD, Wilton P. General practice fundholding: progress to date. *British Journal of General Practice* 1998;48)430:1253–1257

22 Douglas HR, Humphrey C, Lloyd M, Prescott K, Haines A, Rosenthal J, Watt I. Promoting clinical effective practice. Attitudes of fundholding general practitioners to the role of commissioning. *J Manag Med* 1997;11(1):26–34

23 Greener I, Mannion R. Does practice based commissioning avoid the problems of fundholding? *BMJ* 2006;333:1168

24 McCartney M. Farewell Doctor Finlay (radio programme). *BBC Radio 4*, 8 July 2016

25 Kay A. *The Dynamics of Public Policy: Theory and Evidence.* Cheltenham: Edgar Elgar Publishing, 2006, p117

26 Mannion R. General practitioner commissioning in the English National Health Service: continuity, change, and future challenges. *J Health Serv* 2008;38(4):717–30

27 Greener I, Mannion R. Does practice based commissioning avoid the problems of fundholding? (see 23).

28 Smith J, Dixon J, Mays N, McLeod H, Goodwin N, McClelland S, Lewis R, Wyke S, et al. Practice based commissioning: applying the research evidence. *BMJ* 2005;331:1397

29 Lewis R, Curry N, Dixon M. *Practice-based Commissioning: From good idea to effective practice.* London: The King's Fund, May 2007

30 Heron C, Campbell F for Centre for Public Scrutiny. *Practice based commissioning in the NHS: A guide for overview and scrutiny committees.* London: CfPS, March 2010

31 Propper C, Burgess S, Green K. Does Competition between Hospitals Improve the Quality of Care? Hospital Death Rates and the NHS Internal Market. Bristol: University

References

of Bristol, December 2000 (revised February 2002)

32 Street A, et al. Are English treatment centres treating less complex patients? *Health Policy*;94(2):150–157

33 House of Commons Health Committee. *Public Expenditure on Health and Personal Social Services 2007*. London: The Stationary Office, 16 November 2007

34 House of Commons Health Committee. *Independent Sector Treatment Centres: Fourth Report of Session 2005–06: Volume I*. London: The Stationary Office, 25 July 2006

35 Slater E. NHS Reforms Examined: £500m paid in botched NHS contracts to private companies. *Bureau of Investigative Journalism*, 25 May 2011

36 Chard J, Kuczawski M, Black N, van der Meulen J. Outcomes of elective surgery undertaken in independent sector treatment centres and NHS providers in England: audit of patient outcomes in surgery. *BMJ* 2011;343:d6404

37 Bardsley M, Dixon J. Quality of care in independent sector treatment centres. *BMJ* 2011;343:d6936

38 Oussedik S, Haddad F from University College Hospital, London. Further doubts over the performance of treatment centres in providing elective orthopaedic surgery. *J Bone Joint Surg [Br]* 2009;91-B:1125–6

39 Timmins N, ed. Challenges of private provision in the NHS. *BMJ* 2005;331:1193

40 House of Commons Health Committee. *Independent Sector Treatment Centres*. (see 34)

41 House of Commons Health Committee Fourth Report Commissioning, 18 March 2010

42 NHS England. *General Practice Forward View*, April 2016

43 McCartney M. How to misspend £2.4bn. *BMJ* 2016;353:i2366

44 Scottish Government. Integration of Health and Social Care

45 Robertson H for Royal College of Nursing Scotland. *Integration of health and social care: A review of literature and models, Implications for Scotland*. RCN Scotland, January 2011

46 Institute of Public Care at Oxford Brookes University. *Evidence Review: Integrated Health and Social Care – Executive Summary*. Skills for Care, June 2013

47 Pritchard C, Wallace MS. Comparing the USA, UK and 17 Western countries' efficiency and effectiveness in reducing mortality. *J R Soc Med Sh Rep* 2011;2:50

48 Consumer Reports. Why is health care so expensive? *consumerreports.org*, September 2014

49 Commonwealth Fund. U.S. Health Care from a Global Perspective

50 Centers for Medicare and Medicaid Services US. *National Health Expenditures 2014 Highlights*

51 Fuchs VR. Why do other rich nations spend so much less on healthcare? *Atlantic*, 23 July 2014

52 Obama Care Facts. Health Care Facts: Why We Need Health Care Reform

53 OECD Health Statistics 2014: How does the United States compare?

54 International Federation of Health Plans. 2013 Comparative Price Report: Variation in Medical and Hospital Prices by Country

55 Warren E. *Medical Bankruptcy in the United States* featuring article by Himmelstein DU, Thorne D, Woolhandler S, Warren E. Medical Bankruptcy in the United States 2007: Results of a National Survey. *Am J Med* March 2009

56 Austin DA. Medical debt as a cause of consumer bankruptcy. *Marine Law Review* 2014;67(1):1–23

57 Consumer Reports. About the Choosing Wisely campaign

58 David Owen: Health care can never be only a market commodity. *Yorkshire Post*, 5 April 2011

59 Arrow KJ. Uncertainty and the welfare economics of medical care. *American Economic Review* December 1963;LIII(5):941–973

60 Capretta JC, Dayaratna KD. Compelling Evidence Makes the Case for a Market-Driven Health Care System. United States: The Heritage Foundation, 20 December 2013

61 Dowler C. Price competition could raise death rates, experts warn. *HSJ*, 17 December

2010

62 Department of Health White Paper: NHS Confederation response to regulating healthcare providers. NHS Confederation, 11 October 2010. Available at www.nhsconfed.org/~/media/Confederation/Files/public%20access/Response%20to%20Regulating%20healthcare%20providers%20FINAL.pdf.

63 Griffiths R, Bett M, Blyth J, Bailey B. Inquiry to Rt Hon Norman Fowler MP, Secretary of State for Social Services, regarding NHS management. Available at www.nhshistory.net/griffiths.html.

64 Lord Rose for Department of Health. *Leadership for Tomorrow*. London: The Stationary Office, June 2015

65 Lawson N. *The View from No. 11*, p618. (see 19).

66 Timmins, N, Davies E. Glaziers and window breakers: the role of the Secretary of State for Health, in their own words. The HealthFioundation, May 2015

67 Secretary of State for Health. *Equity and Excellence: Liberating the NHS*. London: The Stationary Office, July 2010

68 Gridley K, Spiers G, Aspinal F, Bernard S, Atkin K, Parker G. Can general practitioner commissioning deliver equity and excellence? Evidence from two studies of service improvement in the English NHS. *J Health Services Research &* Policy;17(2):87–93

69 Raffish, J. Revealed: One in five GPs on CCG boards has financial interest in a current provider. *pulsetoday.co.uk*, 23 September 2013

70 Smyth C. Gas and power markets are a 'model for the health service'. *Times*, 25 February 2011

71 House of Commons Health Committee. Commissioning: Further issues: Fifth Report of Session 2010–11. Volume II. London: The Stationary Office, 5 April 2011

72 Hempsons. *Cooperation and Competition: A Step Guide for Foundation Trusts and NHS Trusts*

73 Neville S. NHS chief more willing to embrace competition, says regulator. *Financial Times*, 28 April 2014

74 Secretary of State for Health. *Equity and Excellence: Liberating the NHS*. (see 67).

75 Lind S. GP practices set to be rated out of five stars on 'TripAdvisor-style' websites. *pulsetoday.co.uk*, 16 July 2014

76 Adams S. Now GPs who fail older patients will get 'red warning': Ministers want to reveal how good or bad doctors are at keeping over-60s out of hospital. *Mail on Sunday*, 12 July 2014

77 McLean G, Guthrie B, Mercer SW, Watt GCM. General practice funding underpins the persistence of the inverse care law: cross-sectional study in Scotland. *Br J Gen Pract* 1 December 2015

78 Relph S. How good is your doctor's surgery? Check using this new online service. *Mirror*, 18 November 2014

79 Campbell J, Smith P, Nissen S, Bower P, Elliott M, Roland M. The GP Patient Survey for use in primary care in the National Health Service in the UK — development and psychometric characteristics. *BMC Family Practice* 2009;10:57

80 Coulter A. *Evidence on the effectiveness of strategies to improve patients' experience of cancer care*. Picker Institute, June 2007

81 NHS England. GP patient survey: See how your GP practice is doing or compare practices

82 Al-Abri R, Al-Balushi A. Patient satisfaction survey as a tool towards quality improvement. *Oman Medical Journal* 2014;29(1):3–7

83 Verhoef LM, Van de Belt TH, Engelen LJ, Schoonhoven L, Kool RB. Social media and rating sites as tools to understanding quality of care: a scooping review. Eysenbach G. ed. *Journal of Medical Internet Research* 2014;16(2):e56

84 Moorhead SA, Hazlett DE, Harrison L, Carroll JK, Irwin A, Hoving C. A new dimension of health care: systematic review of the uses, benefits, and limitations of social media for health communication. *J Med Internet Res* 23 April 2013;15(4):e85

References

85 Falkenberg K. Why Rating Your Doctor Is Bad for Your Health. *Forbes*, 21 January 2013

86 Ashworth M, White P, Jongsma H, Schofield P, Armstrong D. Antibiotic prescribing and patient satisfaction in primary care in England: cross-sectional analysis of national patient survey data and prescribing data. *Br J Gen Pract* 7 December 2015
    Kirkwood G, Pollock AM. Patient choice and private provision decreased public provision and increased inequalities in Scotland: a case study of elective hip arthroplasty. *J Pub Health* 28 July 2016

87 Boffey D, Helm T. David Cameron's adviser says health reform is a chance to make big profits. *Guardian*, 14 May 2011

88 Doward J. Calls for greater disclosure on NHS chiefs' meetings with private US health insurer. *Guardian*, 30 August 2014

89 Helm T. Shirley Williams plunges NHS reforms into fresh turmoil. *Guardian*, 3 September 2011

90 NHS England Supply Chain Partners, 27 April 2015 and Doward J. Fears grow over 'land grab' of NHS by private suppliers. *Guardian*, 2 May 2015

91 PricewaterhouseCoopers for Department of Health. *A review of the potential benefits from the better use of information and technology in Health and Social Care: Final report.* London: PWC, 14 January 2013

92 McCartney M. Price Waterhouse Coopers report on technology was expensive and is flawed (blog)

93 McKinsey and Co. Achieving World Class Productivity in the NHS 2009/10 — 2013/14: Detailing the Size of the Opportunity. Department of Health, May 2010

94 Lacobucci G. Dozens of consortia turn to McKinsey. *pulsetoday.co.uk*, 9 March 2011

95 Campbell D. Management consultants get £7m to give GPs business skills. *Guardian*, 12 January 2012

96 Clover B. Barts pays management consultant £1m in 10 months. *HSJ*, 6 October 2014

97 David O. Stop wasting taxpayers' money on management consultancy for the NHS. *BMJ* 2014;349:G7243

98 Rose D. The firm that hijacked the NHS: MoS investigation reveals extraordinary extent of interenational management consultant's role in Lansley's health reforms. *Mail on Sunday*, 12 February 2012

99 Exclusive: NHS regulator spends 40% of budget on consultants. *Yorkshire Post*, 3 May 2013

100 Lacobucci G. Former health secretary takes on another advisory role in private health sector. *BMJ* 17 November 2015;351:h6201

101 Syal R, Hughes S. Ex-health secretary Andrew Lansley to advise firms on healthcare reforms. *Guardian*, 20 October 2015

102 NHS England. Who's Who — the NHS England board

103 Cambridgeshire and Peterborough Clinical Commissioning Group. Ten organisations go through to next stage of integrated Older People's services procurement. *cambridgeshirenadpeterboughccg.nhs.uk*, 9 September 2013

104 KPMG. Stephen Dorrell, Healthcare and Public Sector Advisor to KPMG in the UK.

105 Mathiason N. Labour gets into bed with private medicine. *Guardian*, 19 November 2000

106 Davies H. Company owned by Alan Milburn had £663,000 profit increase in 2013–14. *Guardian*, 29 January 2015

107 Bloomberg. Markets: Stocks

108 PricewaterhouseCoopers: Meet the Team

109 Bridgepoint: Our Team: Alan Milburn

110 Curtis P. Former Labour ministers rushing to take private sector jobs, report finds. *Guardian*, 17 May 2011

111 Articles from Lord Hutton of Furness on Red Blog and Circle Holdings Board of Directors

112 Blackhurst D. PM challenged to clarify Malcolm Rifkind's involvement in £80m NHS deal. *Sentinel*, 25 February 2015

113 Campbell D. NHS being 'atomised' by expansion of private sector's role, say doctors. *Guardian*, 6 January 2013

114 Lacobucci G. A third of NHS contracts awarded since health act have gone to private sector, *BMJ* investigation shows. *BMJ* 2014;314:G7606

115 Craig E. Reality Check: Can we trust NHS privatisation statistics? *BBC*, 30 April 2015

116 House of Commons Health debate, 7 July 2015. Available at hansard.digiminster.com/Commons/2015-07-07/debates/15070743000028/TopicalQuestions.

117 Meek J. It's already happened. *London Review of Books* 22 September 2011;33(18):3–10

118 BASHH Clinical Governance Committee on behalf of BASHH andIndependent Advisory Group on Sexual Health and HIV. *The Experience of Tendering of Sexual Health Services in England as Reported by Genitourinary Medicine Physicians*. BASHH, 12 August 2008

119 Watt N, Campbell D, Farrell S. Circle in talks to exit private contract to run Hinchingbrooke hospital. *Guardian*, 9 January 2015 and Commons Select Committee. Circle's withdrawal from Hinchingbrooke Hospital update report published. *parliament.uk*, 18 March 2015

120 Barrett H. Circle 'bemused' over finance crisis claims relating to Hinchingbrooke Hospital in Huntington. *Hunts Post*, 15 November 2014

121 Commons Select Committee. An update on Hinchingbrooke Hospital Health Care NHS Trust, 2010

122 Commons Select Committee. Circle's withdrawal from Hinchingbrooke Hospital update report published. *parliament.uk*, 18 March 2015

123 Neville S, Plimmer G. NHS group wins biggest patient services tender. *Financial Times*, 1 October 2014

124 Plimmer G. Cambridgeshire healthcare contract hit by exodus of bidders. *Financial Times*, 9 March 2014

125 Ibid.

126 Plimmer G. Collapse of £1.2bn NHS contract raises tendering questions. *Financial Times*, 4 October 2015

127 Perkins A. NHS watchdog signed off doomed £750m contract despite doubts. *Guardian*, 26 January 2016

128 Comptroller and Auditor General, National Audit Office. *Investigation into the collapse of the UnitingCare Partnership contract in Cambridgeshire and Peterborough*. London: The Stationary Office, 14 July 2016

129 Comptroller and Auditor General, National Audit Office. *Memorandum on the provision of the out-of-hours GP service in Cornwall*. London: The Stationary Office, 6 March 2013

130 Serco Cornwall out-of-hours GP contract to end early. *BBC*, 13 December 2013

131 Rise in Mitie service failures at Royal Cornwall Hospitals Trust. *BBC*, 28 July 2015

132 Barton L. Private firm who won NHS contract 'have cut corners'. *Western Morning News*, 22 October 2014

133 Whittell R, Dugan E. Exclusive: Services provider established by outsourcing giant Serco overcharged NHS by millions.   *Independent*, 27 August 2014

134 The next Serco scandal: overcharging the NHS. *corporatewatch.org*, 28 August 2014

135 Stoke NHS hospital scanning contract won by private firm. *Sentinel*, 8 December 2014

136 Tweet by Margaret Hodge

137 Rose J. The Practice: About US

138 Vowles N. John Lewis arrival sealed the end for GP firm as it walks away from contract and 11,500 patients. *The Argus*,   18 January 2016

139 Virgin Care www.virgincare.co.uk/our-values/

140 Boffey D. Virgin Care among firms with lucrative NHS deals and a tax haven status. *Guardian*, 21 March 2015

141 Virgin Care and Freedom of Information requests response to 'Will Virgin Care be open to Freedom of Information requests?

References

142 Sanders M. Getting Rich on the NHS — Reporter Feature. *Channel 4 News*, 5 July 2013

143 Exclusive: Virgin pulls out of Whitby hospital deal. *North Yorks Enquirer*, 24 September 2015

144 Stirling A, Kenny C. Local enhanced services worth millions to be opened up to competition from April. *pulsetoday.co.uk*, 3 January 2014

145 Lister L. In defiance of the evidence. *International Journal of Health Services* 2012;42(1):137–155.

146 Supply Management. 85 per cent of GPs admit they lack commissioning skills. *cips.org*, 4 November 2011

147 Millett D. Exclusive: Obese patients denied surgery by NHS rationing. *gponline.com*, 10 June 2015

148 Campbell D. NHS to 'extend rationing' of healthcare in bid to balance books. *Guardian*, 21 April 2015

149 Burns C. Serco 'looking to offload out-of-hours GP services' in Cornwall. *West Briton*, 13 October 2013

150 Chick C. GPs take over Cornwall's out-of-hours service. *West Briton*, 1 June 2015

151 Lawrence F. Cornish complaints raise questions over national drive to outsource NHS care. *Guardian*, 25 May 2012

152 Bawden A, Campbell D. Out of hours, out of GPs' hands. *Guardian*, 4 June 2013

153 Bartholomew E. Hackney GPs oust Harmoni from out of hours contract. *Hackney Gazette*, 1 October 2013

154 NHS 111 — A Bad Call? (radio programme). *BBC Radio 4*, 18 August 2013

156 Lind S. Rise in A&E attendances caused by NHS 111, emergency medicine leader claims. *pulsetoday.co.uk*, 14 January 2015 and Turner J, O'Cathain A, Knowles E, Nicholl J. Impact of the urgent care telephone service NHS 111 pilot sites: a controlled before and after study. *BMJ Open* 2013;3:e0003451

157 Roberts N. Exclusive: NHS 111 risks 'were known before launch'. *gponline.com*, 5 July 2013 and Calkin S. NHS Direct nurses stage a 'work in' protest. *Nursing Times*, 2 May 2012

158 Torjesen I. NHS Direct backs out of contracts to run NHS 111 because of poor funding *BMJ* 2013;347:f4837

159 *Channel 4 News*, www.channel4.com/programmes/dispatches/articles/2013/undercover-in-nhs-111/738

160 Lacobucci G. The battle for NHS 111: who should run it now? *BMJ* 2014;348:f7659

161 Ebell MH, Lundgren J, Youngpairoj S. How long does a cough last? Comparing patients' expectations with data from a systematic review of the literature. *Ann Fam Med* January/February 2013;11(1):5–13 162Turner J, et al. Impact of the urgent care telephone service NHS 111 pilot sites: a controlled before and after study. (see 155).

162 Royal College of General Practitioners. *The 2022 GP Compendium of Evidence*. London: Royal College of General Practitioners, 20 May 2013

163 Saultz JW, Albedaiwi W. Interpersonal Continuity of Care and Patient Satisfaction: A Critical Review. *Annals of Family Medicine* 2004;2(5):445–451and Freeman G, Hughes J. *Continuity of care and the patient experience*. London: The King's Fund, 2010

164 Björkelund C, Maun A, et al. Impact of continuity on quality of primary care: from the perspective of citizens' preferences and multi morbidity — position paper of the European Forum for Primary Care. *Quality in Primary Care* 2013;21:193–204

165 Saultz JW, Lochner J. Interpersonal Continuity of Care and Care Outcomes: A Critical Review. *Ann Fam Med* March/April 2005;3(2):159–166

166 Chauhan M, Bankart MJ, Labeit A, Baker R. Characteristics of general practices associated with numbers of elective admissions. *J Public Health* December 2012;34(4):584–90

167 National Health Service. Specification for a directed enhanced service: Access to general medical services

168 GP surgeries are 'cheating' the 48-hour access target. *Scotsman*, 26 February 2006

(updated 15 March 2006)

169 Silver L. GP Business: Achieving access targets. *gponline.com*, 1 March 2004

170 GP surgeries are 'cheating' the 48-hour access target. *Scotsman*. (see 167).

171 Blair promises action on GP row. *BBC*, 29 April 2005

172 Donnelly L. Ambulances referred by NHS 111 service deliberately delayed under secret trust policy, inquiry finds. *Telegraph*, 28 February 2016

173 Timmins N. MPs warn on scale of NHS efficiency drive. *Financial Times*, 13 December 2010

174 image.guardian.co.uk/sys-files/Society/documents/2004/11/24/PFI.pdf.

175 Pollock AM. PFI and the National Health Service in England. *allysonpollock.com*, June 2013

176 Ibid

177 Gaffney D, Pollock AM, Price D, Shaoul J. NHS capital expenditure and the private finance initiative — expansion or contraction? *BMJ* 1999;319(7201):48–51

178 Comptroller and Auditor General, National Audit Office. *The performance and management of hospital PFI contracts*. London: The Stationary Office, 15 June 2010

179 Treasury Select Committee. Private Finance Initiative: Conclusions and recommendations, 18 July 2011

180 Plimmer G, Neville S. NHS trust becomes first to buy out its PFI contract. *Financial Times*, 1 October 2014

181 Plimmer G. NHS hospital trust seeks private help. *Financial Times*, 7 April 2014

182 Medick R, Donnelly L, Kirk A. The PFI hospitals costing NHS £2bn every year. *Telegraph*, 18 July 2015

183 Gaffney D, Pollock AM, Price D, Shaoul J. PFI in the NHS — is there an economic case? *BMJ* 1999;319:116

184 Nuffield Trust. *Feeling the crunch: NHS finances to 2020*. London: Nuffield Trust, 2016

185 Donnelly L. The list of 66 A&E and maternity units being hit by cuts. *Telegraph*, 26 October 2014

186 Kenney C, Kaffash J, Matthews-King A. Revealed: Sixty GP practices across the country facing imminent closure. *pulsetoday.co.uk*, 3 July 2014

187 Price C. CCG backs down on plan to block all non-urgent GP referrals. *pulsetoday.co.uk*, 11 August 2016

188 Carrell S. Scottish NHS left needing 'fundamental changes' after budget cuts, says report. *Guardian*, 22 October 2015

189 Lind S. GPs to be given rationing thresholds for surgery. *pulsetoday.co.uk*, 15 January 2013

CHAPTER 7

1 House of Commons Health Committee. *Modernising Medical Careers: Third Report of Session 2007–08: Volume I*. London: The Stationary Office, 24 April 2008

2 Gaines S. Training overhaul blamed for junior doctors fiasco. *Guardian*, 8 October 2007

3 Hewitt attacked over jobs website. *BBC*, 1 May 2007

4 Tooke J, et al. Aspiring to Excellence: *Final Report of the Independent Inquiry into Modernising Medical Careers*. London: MMC Inquiry, 2008

5 Charlton R. Revalidation: Gaining CPD Credits. *gponline.com*, 23 September 2010

6 Critchley R, Ader P, Godden A, Ball K for NHS Revalidation Support Team. *The Early Benefits and Impact of Medical Revalidation: Report on research findings in year one*.

7 General Medical Council. Patient Questionnaire form

8 Archer J, Regan de Bere S, Bryce M, Nunn S, Lynn N, Coombes L, Roberts M. *Understanding the rise in Fitness to Practise complaints from members of the public*. Plymouth: Plymouth University Peninsula Schools of Medicine & Dentistry, 30 January 2014

9 British Medical Association. BMA quarterly tracker survey, Current views from across the medical profession, Quarter 2: April 2015

References

10 Lind S. GP vacancy rate at highest ever, with 50% rise in empty posts. *pulsetoday.co.uk*, 29 April 2015

11 Hughes D, Clarke V. Thousands of NHS nursing and doctor posts lie vacant. *BBC*, 29 February 2016

12 Bourne T, Vanderhaegen J, Vranken R, Wynants L, De Cock B, Peters M, Timmerman D, Van Calster B, Jaimbrant M, Van Audenhove C. Doctors' experiences and their perception of the most stressful aspects of complaints processes in the UK: an analysis of qualitative survey data. *BMJ Open* 2016;6(7):e011711

13 McGivern G, Fischer MD. Medical Regulation, Spectacular Transparency and the Blame Business. Author's version of paper published in *J Health Organization and Management* 2010;24(6):597–610

14 Eaton L. BMA calls for investigation into cost of MTAS. *BMJ* 2007;335:534

15 House of Commons Debate on Liver Diseases: Alcoholic Drinks, 13 March 2007 Daily Hansard written answers

16 House of Commons debate record, 6 June 2007

17 Oates J. NHS IT: What went wrong, what will go wrong. *Register*, 30 May 2008

18 Bowers S. Where the NHS's software scheme went wrong. *Guardian*, 21 March 2010

19 House of Commons Public Accounts. The Dismantled National Programme for IT in the NHS — Public Accounts Committee Conclusions and recommendations

20 Duffin C. GPs can only refer via Choose and Book, CCG rules. *pulsetoday.co.uk*, 10 April 2015

21 Matthews-King A. GPs must offer more choice for outpatient referrals, Monitor says. *pulsetoday.co.uk*, 7 August 2014

22   Matthews-King A. GPs may face penalties for not using new-look Choose and Book for referrals. *pulsetoday.co.uk*, 13 February 2014

23 Health & Social Care Information Centre. NHS e-Referral Service: Realising the Benefits

24 Modayil PC, Hornigold R, Glore RJ, Bowdler DA. Patients' attendance at clinics is worse with choose and book. *BMJ* 2009;338:b396

25 Greenhalgh T, Stones R, Swinglehurst D. Choose and Book: A sociological analysis of 'resistance' expert system. *Social Science & Medicine* March 2014;104:210–219

26 Scottish Government. Heat Target information

27 Bouamrane M, Mair FS. A qualitative evaluation of general practitioners' views on protocol-driven eRefferal in Scotland. *BMC Medical Informatics and Decision Making* 2014;14(1):1472–6947

28 Scottish Care Information. SCI Store

29 McCartney M. At last, an NHS good news story. *Financial Times*, 29 September 2006

30 Turner N. Renal PatientView: Progress and Plans

31 Davies M, Elwyn G. Referral management centres: promising innovations or Trojan horses? *BMJ* 2006;332:844

32 MDU. Referral management centres FAQs

33 O'Dowd A. GP consortium agrees partnership with private firm to run referral service. *BMJ* 2011;342:c7470

34 Quinn I. Private firm screening GP referrals remotely. *pulsetoday.co.uk*, 2 February 2011

35 GPs axe remote referral gateway run by private firm. *pulsetoday.co.uk*, 2 March 2012

36 Gateways using nurses to screen GP referrals. *pulsetoday.co.uk*, 10 August 2011

37 Kaffash J. GPs to be 'rewarded for cutting down referrals. *pulsetoday.co.uk*, 20 March 2015

38 Cooper R, Sunney W. How peer review reduced GP referrals by 25% in two months. *pulsetoday.co.uk*, 20 March 2012

39 The King's Fund. Referral management centres fail to deliver savings, according to new research from The King's Fund (press release). London: The King's Fund, 12 August 2010

40 Xiang A, Smith H, Hine P, et al. Impact of a referral management "gateway" on the quality of referral letters; a retrospective time series cross sectional review. *BMC Health Services Research* 2013;13:310

41 Blank L, Baxter S, Buckley Woods H, Goyder E, Lee A, Payne N, Rimmer M. Referral interventions from primary to specialist care: a systematic review of international evidence. *B J Gen Pract* December 2014;64(629):e765–e774

42 Cox JMS, Steel N, Clark AB, Kumaravel B, Bachmann MO. Do referral-management schemes reduce hospital outpatient attendances? Time-series evaluation of primary care referral management. *Br J Gen Pract* June 2013; 63(611):e386–e392

43 Ball SL, Greenhaigh J, Roland M. Referral management centres as a means of reducing outpatients attendances: how do they work and what influences successful implementation and perceived effectiveness? *BMC Family Practice* 2016;17(1):1471–2296

44 Hippisley-Cox J, Hardy C, Pringle M, Fielding K, Carlisle R, Chilvers C, et al. The effect of deprivation on variations in general practitioners' referral rates: a cross sectional study of computerised data on new medical and surgical outpatient referrals in Nottinghamshire. *BMJ* 1997;314:1458

45 NHS Scotland. *National Therapeutic Indicators 2014/15*

46 Easton G, Saxena S. Antibiotic prescribing for upper respiratory tract infections in children: how can we improve? *London Journal of Primary Care* 2010;3(1):37–41

47 Albert RK, Connett J, Bailey WC, Casaburi R, et al. Azithromycin for prevention of exacerbations of COPD. *N Engl J Med* 2011;365:689–698

48 Pinder R, Sallis A, Berry D, Chadborn T for Public Health England and Department of Health. *Behaviour change and antibiotic prescribing in healthcare settings: Literature review and behavioural analysis.* London: Public Health England, February 2015

49 Ashworth M, White P, Jongsma H, Schofield P, Armstrong D. Antibiotic prescribing and patient satisfaction in primary care in England: cross-sectional analysis of national patient survey data and prescribing data. *Br J Gen Pract* December 2015

50 Roland M, Elliott M, Lyratzopoulos G, Barbiere J, Parker RA, Smith P, et al. Reliability of patient responses in pay for performance schemes: analysis of national General Practitioner Patient Survey data in England. *BMJ* 2009;339:b3851

51 NHS England. GP patient survey: See how your GP practice is doing or compare practices [gp-patient.co.uk].

52 Hallworth M, et al. Provision of social norm feedback to high prescribers of antibiotics in general practice: a pragmatic national randomised controlled trial. *Lancet*;387(10029):1743–1752

53 Comptroller and auditor general, National Audit Office. T*he Care Quality Commission: Regulating the quality and safety of health and adult social care.* London: The Stationary Office, 2 December 2011

54 Millett D. GPs face seven-fold increase in CQC fees by 2017/18. *gponline.com*, 2 November 2015

55 Kaffash J. Practices to pay almost £2,000 more in CQC fees from April. *pulsetoday.co.uk*, 30 March 2016

56 Care Quality Commission. *Intelligent Monitoring: NHS GP practices: Indicators and methodology.* CQC, November 2014

57 Millet D. Practices labelled 'high risk' by CQC found to be 'good' after inspection. *gponline. com*, 9 January 2015

58 Davis J. Revealed: Hundreds of practices rated risky after CQC botched up patient experience data. *pulsetoday.co.uk*, 17 December 2014

59 Care Quality Commission. Update to GP Intelligent Monitoring. CQC, 27 March 2015

60 Health Group Internal Audit. Heath Group Internal Audit: "Protected Disclousre" in 2014 — Review of two 2013 Care Quality Commission procurements. London: The Stationary Office, June 2015

61 Davis J. CQC trawling through 6,000 comments a month on patient websites. *pulsetoday. co.uk*, 24 July 2015

62 Clark T. New research suggests why general election polls were so inaccurate. *Guardian*, 12 November 2015

63 My CQC inspection was the most unpleasant exercise of my career so far. *pulsetoday.co.uk*,

References

27 May 2014

64 CQC: callous, quarrelsome, crude. *British Medical* Association, 18 March 2016

65 The true cost of a CQC inspection. *pulsetoday.co.uk*, 26 June 2015

66 Lind S. Field: Presentation skills necessary to receive CQC outstanding rating. *pulsetoday. co.uk*, 30 June 2016

67 Ramesh R. CQC publishes suppressed report on Morecambe Bay inspections. *Guardian*, 21 June 2013

68 Donnelly L. Cover-up over hospital scandal at University Hospitals of Morecambe Bay NHS Trust. Telegraph, 18 June 2013

69 Report by the Right Honourable Sir Anthony Hooper to the General Medical Council, 19 March 2015. The Handling by the General Medical Council of Cases Involving Whistleblowers. Available at www.gmc-uk.org/Hooper_review_final_60267393.pdf.

70 Department of Health. *The NHS Plan: A Plan for Investment, a Plan for Reform*. London: The Stationary Office, 2000, p28

71 Bevan G. Regulation and system management in Dixon A, Mays N, Jones L, eds. *Understanding New Labour's Market Reforms of the English NHS*. London: The King's Fund, 2011

72 Healthcare Improvement Scotland. What we do

73 Grol R. Quality improvement by peer review in primary care: a practical guide. *Quality in Health Care* 1994;3L147–152

74 Ball SL, et al. Referral management centres as a means of reducing outpatients attendances (see 43).

CHAPTER 8

1 Osler W. *Aequanimitas: with other addresses to Medical students, Nurses and Practitioners of Medicine*. *The Master-Word in Medicine*. 2nd ed. Philedelphia: P Blakiston Sons & Co, 1910; pp363–389.

2 Galen. *The Best Doctor is also a Philosopher*

3 Fraser Brockington C, Lambert DP. The vocation of medicine. *Lancet* 27 November 1948;252(6535):871–872

4 Ibid.

5 McCartney M. Farewell Doctor Finlay (radio programme). *BBC Radio 4*, 8 July 2016

6 Tudor Hart J. The inverse care law. *Lancet* 27 February 1971;297(7696):405–27. Available at www.sochealth.co.uk/national-health-service/public-health-and-wellbeing/poverty-and-inequality/the-inverse-care-law/

7 Hart JT. Why family doctors should not advertise. *J Royal College Gen Pract* 1988;38(317):559–562

8 Royal College of Obstetricians and Gynaecologists. *Multiple Pregnancy Following Assisted Reproduction*, January 2011. Available at www.rcog.org.uk/globalassets/documents/guidelines/sip_no_22.pdf.

9 Radical Statistics Health Group, In Defence of the National Health Service. *Int J Health Serv* October 1980;10(4):611–645

10 Ibid.

11 Triggle N. Jeremy Hunt: Doctors 'must work weekends'. *BBC*, 16 July 2015

12 Galen. *The Best Doctor* (see 2).

13 Making Britain Better. *BBC*, 1 July 1998

14 Odone, Christine Doctors are no longer gods. Daily Telegraph 19/1/12

15 Berger J. *A Fortunate Man: The Story of a Country Doctor*. London: Allen Lane, 1967, page 70

16 Barsky AJ. Hidden Reasons Some Patients Visit Doctors. *Ann Intern Med* 1981;94:492–498

17 Widgery D. *Some Lives: A GP's East End*. London: Simon and Schuster, 1992 page 236

18 Stevenson AD, Phillips CB, Anderson KJ. Resilience among doctors who work in challenging areas: a qualitative study. *B J Gen Pract* 2011;61(588):e404–e410

19 Heath I. *The Mystery of General Practice*. John Fry Trust Fellowship, 1995

20 O'Riordan M, Skelton J, de la Croix A. Heartlift patients? An interview-based study of GP trainers and the impact of 'patients they like. *Family Practice* 2008;25(5):349–354

21 Kelly Á. Growing up in care. *BMJ* 2016;352:i1085

22 Zsigmond D. GPs' demoralisation is due to our loss of human connection

23 Sandel MJ. *What Money Can't Buy: The Moral Limits of Markets*. London: Penguin, 2013, p202.

24 Nutting PA, Goodwin MA, Flocke SA, Zyzanski SJ, Strange KC. Continuity of primary care: to whom does it matter and when? *Ann Fam Med* 2003;1(3):149–155

25 Sav A, McMillan SS, Kelly F, et al. The ideal healthcare: priorities of people with chronic conditions and their carers. *BMC Health Services Research* 2015;15:551

26 Miedaner F, Allendorf A, Kuntz L, Woopen C, Roth B. The role of nursing team continuity in the treatment of very-low-birth-weight infants: findings from a pilot study. *J Nursing Management* 2016;24(4):458–464

Omer S, Priebe S, Giacco D. Continuity across inpatient and outpatient mental health care or specialisation of teams? A systematic review. *Eur Psychiatry* February 2015;30(2):258–70

Reddy A, Pollack CE, Asch DA, Canamucio A, Werner RM. The effect of primary care provider turnover on patient experience of care and ambulatory quality of care. *JAMA Intern Med* July 2015;175(7):1157–62

Sykes W, Groom C for Equality and Human Rights Commission. *Older people's experiences of home care in England*. Manchester: Equality and Human Rights Commission, 2011

27 Grinberg C, Hawthorne M, LaNoue M, Brenner J, Mautner D. The core of care management: the role of authentic relationships in caring for patients with frequent hospitalizations. *Population Health Management* 2016;19(4):248–256

28 Grant AM, Hofmann DA. It's not all about me: motivating hand hygiene among health care professionals by focusing on patients. *Psychological Science* December 2011

29 Ballatt J, Campling P. *Intelligent Kindness: Reforming the Culture of Healthcare*. London: Royal College of Psychiatrists, June 2011. Available at www.rcpsych.ac.uk/usefulresources/publications/books/rcpp/9781908020048.aspx.

30 Campling P. Reforming the culture of healthcare: the case for intelligent kindness. *B J Psych Bull* February 2015;39(1):1–5

31 Wardrop M. Andrew Lansley: criticism of NHS reforms is 'out of date and unfair'. *Telegraph*, 24 June 2012

32 Dixon-Woods M, Baker R, Charles K, Dawson J, et al. Culture and behaviour in the English National Health Service: overview of lessons from a large multi method study. *BMJ Qual Saf* 2013;4(23):106–15

33 Borrill CS, Carletta J, Carter AJ, Dawson JF, Garrod S, Rees A, Richards A, Shapiro D, West MA. *The Effectiveness of Health Care Teams in the National Health Service*

34 Campbell D. NHS has the west's most stressed GPs, survey reveals. *Guardian*, 19 January 2016

35 Bush M, Seager M. Why public sector workers need a Samaritans-style helpline. *Guardian*, 22 June 2015

36 Shanafelt, Tait D. et al. Relationship Between Clerical Burden and Characteristics of the Electronic Environment With Physician Burnout and Professional Satisfaction. *Mayo Clinic Proceedings* July 2016;91(7):836-848

37 NHS Online. Number of written complaints about NHS falls by 4 per cent, 15 September 2016

38 Horsfall S for General Medical Council. *Doctors who commit suicide while under GMC fitness to practise investigation: Internal review*. London: GMC, 2014

39 Bourne T, Wynants L, Peters M, Van Audenhove C, Timmerman D, Van Calster B, Jalmbrant M. Health policy — Research:
The impact of complaints procedures on the welfare, health and clinical practise of 7926 doctors in the UK: a cross-sectional survey. *BMJ Open* 2015;5(1):e006687.

40 Menzies Lyth I. Social Systems as a Defense Against Anxiety: An Empirical Study of the

References

Nursing Service of a General Hospital. *Dynamics of Organizational Change*, p439–462

41 Redinbaugh EM, Sullivan AM, Block SD, Gadmer NM, Lakoma M, Mitchell AM, et al. Doctors' emotional reactions to recent death of a patient: cross sectional study of hospital doctors. *BMJ* 2003;327:185

42 Trufelli DC, Bensi CG, Garcia JB, Narahara JL, Abrão MN, Diniz RW, Miranda Vda C, Soares HP, Del Giglio A. Burnout in cancer professionals: a systematic review and meta-analysis. *Eur J Cancer Care (Engl)* November 2008;17(6):524–31

Orton P, Orton C, Pereira Gray D. Depersonalised doctors: a cross-sectional study of 564 doctors, 760 consultations and 1876 patient reports in UK general practice. *BMJ Open* 2012;2:e000274 and Wurm W, Vogel K, Holl A, Ebner C, Bayer D, Mörkl S, Szilagyi IS, Hotter E, Kapfhammer HP, Hofmann P. Depression-Burnout Overlap in Physicians. *PLoS One* March 2016 March;11(3):e0149913

43 T D Wall, R I Bolden, C S Borrill, A J Carter, D A Golya, G E Hardy, C E Haynes, J E Rick, D A Shapiro, M A West. Minor psychiatric disorder in NHS trust staff: occupational and gender differences. *B J Psych* December 1997;171(6):519–523

44 West M, Dawson J. *NHS Staff Management and Health Service Quality*

45 McCabe S. Where have we gone wrong? *B J Gen Pract* 2013;63(606):35

46 Longmore JM, Wilkinson IB, Rajagopalan SR. *Oxford Handbook of Clinical Medicine*. Oxford: Oxford University Press, 2004

47 Schwingshackl A. The fallacy of chasing after work-life balance. *Frontiers in Pediatrics* 2014;2: 2296–2360

48 Cooper C. Medical union to seek legal advice on treatment of young doctors amid fear NHS is breaching Human Rights Act. *Independent*, 15 May 2015

49 European Working Time Directive: Junior doctor rota gaps. *BMA*, 30 June 2016

50 Elgot J. Junior doctors will boycott review into poor morale. *Guardian*, 26 February 2016

51 James Lind Alliance: History

52 NHS England. Safe Haven Cafe in Aldershot

53 Khan A, Furtak SL, Melvin P, Rogers JE, Schuster MA, Landrigan CP. Parent-Reported Errors and Adverse Events in Hospitalized Children. *JAMA Pediatr* 2016;170(4):e154608

54 Snow R, Fulop N. Understanding issues associated with attending a young adult diabetes clinic: a case study. Diabetic Medicine. 2012;29(2):257–259

55 National Institute for Health and Care Excellence. Cardiovascular disease: risk assessment and reduction, including lipid modification, NICE, July 2014 (updated September 2016)

56 Fontana F, Perviz Asaria, Michela Moraldo, Judith Finegold, Khalil Hassanally, Charlotte H. Manisty and Darrel P. Francis, Patient-Accessible Tool for Shared Decision Making in Cardiovascular Primary Prevention: Balancing Longevity Benefits Against Medication Disutility. *Circulation* 17 June 2014;129(24)

57 Frosch DL, Kaplan RM. Shared decision making in clinical medicine: past research and future directions. *Am J Prev Med* 1999;17(4):285–294

58 Coxeter P, Del Mar CB, McGregor L, Beller EM, Hoffmann TC. Interventions to facilitate shared decision making to address antibiotic use for acute respiratory infections in primary care. *Cochrane Database of Systematic Reviews* 2015;11:CD010907

59 Costelloe C, Metcalfe C, Lovering A, Mant D, Hay AD. Effect of antibiotic prescribing in primary care on antimicrobial resistance in individual patients: systematic review and meta-analysis. *BMJ* 2010;340:c2096

60 Stacey D, Légaré F, Col NF, Bennett CL, Barry MJ, Eden KB, Holmes-Rovner M, Llewellyn-Thomas H, Lyddiatt A, Thomson R, Trevena L, Wu JH. Decision aids for people facing health treatment or screening decisions. *Cochrane Database Syst Rev* 28 January 2014;1:CD001431

61 Veroff D, Marr A, Wennberg DE. Enhanced support for shared decision making reduced costs of care for patients with preference-sensitive conditions. *Health Aff (Millwood)* February 2013;32(2):285–93

62 Walsh T, Barr PJ, Thompson R, Ozanne E, O'Neill C, Elwyn G. Undetermined impact of patient decision support interventions on healthcare costs and savings: systematic review.

BMJ 23 January 2014;348:g188

63 Teaster PB, O'Brien JG. The elder mistreatment of overtreatment at end of life. *Public Policy Aging Report* 2014;24(3):92–96

64 Periyakoil VS, Neri E, Fong A, Kraemer H. Do Unto Others: Doctors' Personal End-of-Life Resuscitation Preferences and Their Attitudes toward Advance Directives. *PLoS ONE* 2014;9(5):e98246

CHAPTER 9

1 Schünemann HJ, Moja L. Reviews: Rapid! Rapid! Rapid! …and systematic. *Systematic Reviews* 2015;4(4):046–4053

2 Whitty CMJ. What makes an academic paper useful for health policy? *BMC Medicine* 2015;13(1):1741–7015

3 Cairney P. *The Politics of Evidence-Based Policy Making*. London: Palgrave Macmillan, 2016.

4 Alliance for Useful Evidence

5 History and Policy. Who We Are

6 Center for Evidence-based Policy

7 Grattan Institute. GPs and Primary Care

8 Campbell Collaboration

9 Goldacre B. *Building Evidence into Education*. Department of Education, March 2013. Available at www.gov.uk/government/news/building-evidence-into-education.

10 Katikireddi SV, Higgins M, Bond L, Bonell C, Macintyre S. How evidence based is English public health policy? *BMJ* 2011;343:d7310

11 Rutter J, Gold J. *Show Your Workings: Assessing How Government Uses Evidence to Make Policy*. London: Institute for Government, October 2015

12 Barton T, Lewis C. England NHS multimillion-pound contract consultants axed. *BBC*, 21 July 2016

13 Buchanan M. Southern Health NHS Trust 'paid millions' to Katrina Percy's associates. *BBC*, 29 July 2016

14 Comptroller and Auditor General, National Audit Office for Department of Health and NHS England. Investigation into the Cancer Drugs Fund. London: National Audit Office, 16 September 2015

15 Ashworth M, Marshall M. Financial incentives and professionalism: another fine mess. *B J Gen Pract* 2015;65(637): 394–395

16 Rutter J, Gold J. *Show Your Workings: Assessing How Government Uses Evidence to Make Policy*. (see 11).

17 Glass C, Knight R, Zyada A. Written evidence from Cass Business School regarding junior doctors and management of NHS clinical staff numbers in response to National Audit Office report. London: City University London

18 Ibid.

19 Campbell D, Travis A. Junior doctors row has derailed seven-day NHS plans, says top doctor. *Guardian*, 24 March 2016

20 London School of Economics and Political Science. Bad science concerning NHS competition is being used to support the controversial Health and Social Care Bill

21 Socialist Health Association. Bevan's speech to the Royal Medico-Psychological Association, 5 September 1945

22 Pope C. Heidi Alexander brokers cross-party plan with doctors' backing to call off strike. *Labour List*, 24 April 2016

23 Junior doctors' strikes: Jeremy Hunt rejects plan to pilot contract. *BBC*, 24 April 2016

24 www.abpi.org.uk/our-work/disclosure/Pages/DocumentLibrary.aspx

25 Muirhead C. Dr Mark Taylor Psychiatrist at RCPsychScot meeting, 29Jan16 (YouTube Video)

26 Heighton L, Malnick E, Newell C, Telford L, Fayaz S. Lavish trips laid on by drugs firms to 'sway' NHS staff. *Telegraph*, 22 July 2015 and Heighton L, Malnick E, Newell C, Telford

References

L, Fayaz S. NHS bosses paid by drug firms. *Telegraph*, 22 July 2016

27 Dodge I for NHS England. Mananging conflicts of interest (Paper: PB.31.03.2016/09). NHS England, 2016

28 McCartney M. Partnerships: pharma is closer than you think. *BMJ* 2015;351:h3688

29 Ornstein C, Grochowski Jones R, Tigas M. Now There's Proof: Docs Who Get Company Cash Tend to Prescribe More Brand-Name Meds. *ProPublica*, 17 March 2016

30 National Institute for Health and Care Excellence. Behind the Headlines: Is NICE influenced by pharma? NICE, 12 March 2014

31 McCartney M. Partnerships: pharma is closer than you think. (see 28).

32 The King's Fund. The NHS in a nutshell: Health care spending compared to other countries

33 The King's Fund. NHS trusts' deficit estimated at £2.3 billion as NHS financial crisis deepens (press release), 18 February 2016

34 House of Commons Health Committee. *Impact of the Spending Review on health and social care*. Available at www.publications.parliament.uk/pa/cm201617/cmselect/cmhealth/139/13904.htm.

35 NHS England. Five Year Forward View. NHS England, October 2014

36 House of Commons Public Accounts Committee. Sustainability and financial performance of acute hospital trusts, 10 March 2016. Available at www.publications.parliament.uk/pa/cm201516/cmselect/cmpubacc/709/70906.htm.

37 Merrifield N. Trusts told to fill only 'essential' vacancies by regulator. *Nursing Times*, 4 August 2015

38 West D. Solve deficits and protect patients or face suspension, Hunt warns boards. *HSJ*, 15 January 2016

39 www.health.org.uk/sites/default/files/Spending-Review-Nuffield-Health-Kings-Fund-December-2015_spending_review_what_does_it_mean_for_health_and_social_care.pdf

40 Donnelly L. NHS being pressured by government to "fiddle the figures" to make finances seem better, documents reveal. *Telegraph*, 24 March 2016

41 Campbell D. One in five GP surgeries in London may close within three years. *Guardian*, 13 February 2016

42 Meacock, R, Doran, T, and Sutton, M. What are the Costs and Benefits of Providing Comprehensive Seven-day Services for Emergency Hospital Admissions?. *Health Econ* 2015;24:907–912

43 The King's Fund. The NHS in a nutshell: Health care spending compared to other countries. (see 32).

44 Appleby J, Robertson R, Taylor E. Health. *British Social Attitudes*;32. London: NatCen Social Research

45 Ruotsalainen JH, Verbeek JH, Mariné A, Serra C. Preventing occupational stress in healthcare workers. *Cochrane Database of Systematic Reviews*, 7 April 2015

46 Osaro E, Chima N. Challenges of a negative work load and implications on morale, productivity and quality of service delivered in NHS laboratories in England. *Asian Pacific Journal of Tropical Biomedicine* 2014;4(6):421–429

47 Royal College of Nursing. RCN Policy and International Department Policy Briefing 02/15: The Buurtzorg Nederland (home care provider) model Observations for the United Kingdom (UK). RCN, August 2015

48 Tomlinson J. Lessons from "the other side": teaching and learning from doctors' illness narratives. *BMJ Careers*, 2 June 2014

49 Simple Isn't Easy – changing the way the NHS communicates with patients. *futurepatientblog.com*, 11 January 2016

50 Alison Cameron: Coming out of the box. *BMJ*, 17 July 2014

51 Greenhalgh T, Snow R, Ryan S, Rees S, Salisbury H. Six 'biases' against patients and carers in evidence-based medicine. *BMC Medicine* 2015;13:200

52 Greenhalgh T. Future-proofing relationship-based care: a priority for general practice. *B J Gen Pract*;64(628):580

53 NHS Choices. Vaccinations: Who can have the shingles vaccine?

54 CQC: callous, quarrelsome, crude. *BMA*, 18 March 2016 (updated 30 June 2016)
55 Jeremy Hunt, the Guardian, and the importance of getting the stats right. *understandinguncertainty.org*, 21 November 2015
56 Andrew Lang. Wikiquote
57 Martin GP, McKee L, Dixon-Woods M. Beyond metrics? Utilizing 'soft intelligence' for healthcare quality and safety. *Social Science & Medicine* October 2015;142:19–26
58 Campaign for the NHS Reinstatement Bill
59 Campaign for the NHS Reinstatement Bill. Peter Roderick reflects on what happened to the NHS Bill in the Commons on 11 March 2016
60 Greaves F, Laverty AA, Pape U, et al. Performance of new alternative providers of primary care services in England: an observational study, *J R Soc Med* 2015;108(5):171–183
61 Paton C. At what cost? Paying the price for the market in the English NHS. London: Centre for Health and the Public Interest, February 2014
62 National Institute for Health and Care Excellence. NICE technology appraisal guidance
63 National Institute for Health and Care Excellence. NICE calls for an end to postcode lottery of IVF treatment. NICE, 23 October 2014
64 National Institute for Health and Care Excellence. Safe staffing for nursing in adult inpatient wards in acute hospitals. NICE, July 2014
65 National Institute for Health and Care Excellence. NHS England asks NICE to suspend safe staffing programme. NICE, 4 June 2015
66 National Institute for Health and Care Excellence. NICE releases safe staffing evidence reviews. NICE, 18 January 2016
67 Campbell D. NHS 'backtracking' on ward nurse numbers introduced after Mid Staffs. *Guardian*, 13 October 2015
68 Unison. Unison's staffing levels survey 2015: Red Alert Unsafe Staffing Levels Rising. London: Unison, 2015
69 King's College London. Policy [+] March 2012;34
70 Lintern S. CQC wants 'sophisticated' approach to safe staffing. *Nursing Times*, 29 July 2016
71 Griffiths P, Ball J, Murrells T, Jones S, Rafferty AM. Registered nurse, healthcare support worker, medical staffing levels and mortality in English hospital trusts: a cross-sectional study. *BMJ Open* 2016;6:e008751
72 Cooper C. NHS hospitals told not to fill vacancies as cash crisis bites. *Independent*, 3 August 2015
73 Marangozov R, Williams M, Buchan J. *The labour market for nurses in the UK and its relationship to the demand for, and supply of, international nurses in the NHS: Final Report.* Brighton: Institute for Employment Studies, July 2016
74 Philip K. 15 minutes with… Iona Heath: Seeing people in their own clothes. *BMJ Careers*, 15 June 2011
75 Mathers N, Hodgkin P. The Gatekeeper and the Wizard: a fairy tale. *Br Med J* 1989 (298) 172-3
76 Lafond S, Arora S, Charlesworth A, McKeon A for Nuffield Trust. *Into the Red: The State of the NHS' Finances.* London: Nuffield Trust, July 2014

Index

Index

Index

Index